Social Work
with Immigrants
and Refugees

Social Work
with Immigrants
and Refugees

Angela Shen Ryan, DSW
Editor

The Haworth Press, Inc.
New York • London • Norwood (Australia)

Social Work with Immigrants and Refugees has also been published as *Journal of Multicultural Social Work*, Volume 2, Number 1 1992.

The Haworth Press, Inc., 10 Alice Street, Binghamton, NY 13904-1580, USA

Library of Congress Cataloging-in-Publication Data

Social Work with Immigrants and Refugees / Angela Shen Ryan, editor.
    p. cm.
    "Has also been published as Journal of Multicultural Social Work, volume 2, number 1, 1992"-T.p. verso
    Includes bibliographical references.
    ISBN 1-56024-354-6 (H : Acid Free Paper). –ISBN 1-56024-355-4 (S : Acid Free Paper)
    1. Social work with immigrants-United States. 2. Refugees-Services for-United States.
3. Immigrants-Services for-United States. I. Ryan, Angela Shen..
HV4010.S63 1992
362.84.'00973-dc20   92-32667
                                                                                          CIP

Social Work with Immigrants and Refugees

CONTENTS

ABOUT THE EDITOR

Angela Shen Ryan, DSW, is an Associate Professor of Social Work at Hunter College, City University of New York. She has published articles on topics including ethnicity, cross-cultural counseling, and social work practice with immigrants and refugees. She is a member of the National Association of Social Workers, the Council of Social Work Education, and the New York Coalition of Asian-American Mental Health Professionals.

Social Work
with Immigrants
and Refugees

Preface

Over the past decade, hundreds of thousands of displaced persons in the Soviet Union, East Europe, the Middle East and other regions, and millions of refugees in Africa and Asia have left their countries for security and a better way of life. As political upheaval has swept away Communist government across the region, 1.3 million people have left what used to be the Soviet bloc (Tagliabue, 1991). Tens of thousands of Albanians have fled across the Adriatic to Italy (Cowell, 1991). In both the United States and Canada, the number of refugees from many countries has grown very rapidly, creating new challenges for policy makers and service providers alike.

The numbers alone are staggering, and the impact of new immigrants and refugees on the host countries' economies, and on local communities is overwhelming. There are growing debates over immigration policy in the new Europe, the United States, and most of the industrial countries. The host countries, such as the United States, are already seeing an increased demand for the whole spectrum of medical and social services, from job training to emergency housing (Rohter, 1991). No one knows exactly how extensive the flow of migrants will be in Europe and other continents. But the industrial nations' response has been tighter border controls and stricter visa requirements (Schmidt, 1991). The host societies are fearful not only of the possibly uncontrollable numbers but also of the newcomers who present deep differences in race, culture and religion. In the past, people left their countries and settled close by, but today people must often relocate to distant countries. These people experience painful memories of their past and resettlement problems due to loss of home and family comforts as well as excessive demands for survival in a new society with different values and languages. In the host countries there is often a lot of talk about the subject of immigration, but nothing much is being

xiii

done about it. The scarcity of related literature in major social work periodicals reflects this.

This volume has been prepared for human-service professionals who are seeking to help immigrants and refugees undergoing psychosocial adjustment problems. It provides understanding of the realities of the immigrant and refugee experience: the pain and confusion, the struggles to adjust and the rewards of life in a new land. Writers of this collection contribute their personal and professional competence in this area. Special areas addressed include theoretical considerations, social and political factors facing immigrant groups, adjustment problems relating to specific refugee groups such as Soviet immigrants, management issues in service delivery, and training models for service providers. We hope that this book will generate knowledge and awareness concerning the human service challenges associated with immigrants and refugees.

Angela Shen Ryan

REFERENCES

Cowell, A. (1991, August 11). Crestfallen Albanians speak of death. *The New York Times*, p. 12.
Rohter, L. (1991, August 11). New influx of Cuban refugees is creating strains for Florida. *The New York Times*, p. L7.
Schmidt, W. (1991, November 2). Britain proposes curbs on refugee flow. *The New York Times*, P. L+3.
Tagliabue, J. (1991, August 11). Europeans fleeing West in search of a better life. *The New York Times*, p. 12.

The Application
of Family Systems Theory
to Mental Health Services
for Southeast Asian Refugees

Patricia Kelley

SUMMARY. This paper describes a training project for work with Southeast Asian refugees using an integrated family systems approach. The author has found using a model integrating a structural, strategic, life cycle and Milan systemic therapy helpful at three levels of the project work: consulting with agencies serving the population, training students for this work, and intervening clinically with the refugees themselves.

Over 800,000 Southeast Asian refugees have come into this country since 1975 (U.S. Department of State, 1988), with a peak year in 1979. The severe problems facing these people have been recounted in the literature: the trauma in their countries before coming here, the extreme hardships and sometimes torture involved in leaving and getting here, and the culture shock, racism, and language barriers once they arrived (Hoshino, Bamford, and Du-Bois, 1987). Refugee resettlement programs focused on meeting the immediate needs of these families, but the many problems they faced resulted in a disproportionate number of persons needing

Patricia Kelley, PhD, is Associate Professor at the School of Social Work, University of Iowa, Iowa City, IA 52242.

The author expresses appreciation to the Refugee Service Bureau, Iowa Department of Human Services, for the funding which made this project possible. A version of this paper was presented at the Fifth National Conference on the Transcultural Family, Columbus, OH, November 7, 1989.

1

mental health services (Butcher, Egli, Shiota, & Ben-Porath, 1988). Programs have been established to train mental health professionals and para-professionals in culturally sensitive psychotherapy and counseling (Friedman, Tobin, & Koschmann, 1981; Hoshino et al., 1987; Murphy & Frey, 1988), and they have generally emphasized cultural differences, adding that content onto their existing theoretical frameworks, and they included indigenous helpers in their work (Hoshino et al., 1987).

A POPULATION AT RISK

Now, a decade later, these refugees have settled in, often in the problematic inner city, and often in poverty (Hoshino et al., 1987). They are a population at risk; severe psychiatric problems are found in the refugee population at a much higher rate than the general population (Westermeyer, 1986), and there is a higher incidence of marital and family problems, including family violence (Ben-Porath, 1987; Butcher et al., 1988). Furthermore, the children of these refugees have been found to have more physical and psychological problems which can continue to affect them as adults, and may affect their ability to be effective parents themselves (Ben-Porath, 1987; Charron & Ness, 1981).

More recently, these refugees have begun to be mainstreamed into regular mental health services, rather than being treated in special refugee resettlement programs. General service providers, therefore, need to be trained to work with these people, and treatment models which require less specific cultural knowledge and are easily adapted by mainline therapists need to be identified.

FAMILY SYSTEMS APPROACH

In this paper the efficacy of a family systems approach as a basis for the training and delivery of mental health services for this population is argued and illustrated through a case example. Several related approaches (i.e., structural, strategic, Milan systemic) can be classified under a family systems perspective, for they share common theory and assumptions and can be integrated (Keeney & Ross, 1985; Papp, 1983). A family systems approach can encompass a wide variety of therapeutic interventions, and can be accommodated to the belief system of the client. Rather than adding culturally sensitive material to another approach, whether it is an appropriate fit or not, a family systems perspective is broad enough to be open to cultural differences and yet can offer specific prescriptions for intervention. Furthermore, such an approach does not require a great deal of information regarding each cultural group, which is useful because mainline workers can not be taught all of the cultural norms, since there are differences among the various Southeast Asian cultures (Team Associates, 1980). Some understanding of the culture is helpful, of course.

THE TRAINING PROJECT

While systems approaches have been cited as useful in work with ethnic minorities (Ho, 1987), and work with families has been cited as potentially useful with refugees (Butcher et al., 1988; Hirayama & Cetingok, 1988), a review of the major training programs for mental health refugee assistance programs did not yield any that were specifically based on family systems theory (Deinard, 1988; Hoshino et al., 1987; Jaranson & Bamford, 1987). A pilot project was begun at the University of Iowa in 1987 which explicitly based training and services for refugees around family systems theory. To our knowledge, there were no other such programs at that time.

This training project was begun at the University of Iowa School of Social Work with funding for one year from the Iowa Department of Human Services, Bureau of Refugee Programs, under a Federal Office of Refugee Resettlement discretionary grant. While there were several facets to this program, the focus here is on the clinical training for direct service to refugee families and on the testing of clinical practice theory. The theoretical basis of the school's clinical concentration is family systems, and this grant presented the opportunity to test the applicability of this theory to work with refugee families.

APPLICATION OF SYSTEMS PRACTICE
TO THE REFUGEE POPULATION

Family systems theory is a way of explaining human behavior as that which makes sense in context; that is, the context of the family system as well as the community and larger social systems. Biological, psychological, and social factors are all taken into account, but the focus is more on inter-personal and interactive factors than on intra-psychic factors, and on problem resolution or reduction over uncovering unconscious motives. Interventions are aimed at interrupting negative interactive patterns more than restructuring an individual's personality or mental process. Key concepts in systems practice include the search for strengths in the system and the positive connotation of the intent behind behavior, including symptomatic behavior.

Systems approaches seem especially appropriate for working with Southeast Asian refugees experiencing mental health or family problems because of the emphasis on the family and community over the individual, which matches their cultural belief system (Canda, 1989; Hirayama & Cetingok, 1988). The systemic approaches are generally more short term and problem focused, and are therefore less intrusive and more respectful of the family's need for privacy around other issues which need not be discussed. It has been noted that the non-directive and the uncovering therapies are not useful for this population (Butcher et al., 1988); therefore, this problem focused approach seems appropriate. Some systems' approaches, such as strategic therapy (Haley, 1976) and structural therapy (Minuchin, 1974), emphasize a hierarchical over democratic structure, which is consistent with Southeast Asian cultures. The strategic or structural therapist stays in charge of the sessions, and the parents are expected to be in charge of the children. On the other hand, the Milan systemic therapists (Boscolo, Cecchin, Hoffman & Penn, 1987) place less emphasis on hierarchy. This theoretical debate lays the groundwork for good discussions with trainees.

Assessment is quite different from a systemic perspective than from a medical or psychodynamic model. The focus is on getting a problem definition and then obtaining information around that problem in the context (Papp, 1983). The problem is stated in specific and behavioral terms, how and for whom it is a problem is assessed, and the meaning attached to it is addressed. There are similarities here to behavioral and cognitive therapies, but there is more emphasis on the context, on positive connotation, and on strengths of the system. Thus, psychopathology is not presumed or looked for, and most situations are not viewed in that framework, although severe emotional disturbances are recognized and referrals made when appropriate. This de-emphasis on psychopathology is useful with this population since mental illness is viewed as a disgrace (Butcher et al., 1988).

The methods used in this assessment process are different, too. Psychological tests and mental status exams, which have been questioned for their lack of cultural relevance (Westermeyer, 1986), are not necessary in a systemic assessment. Standard intake questions may not be culturally relevant either. For example, "age" on a child's papers may not be the same as actual age; "religion" presumes that there is one belief whereas some Asians borrow from many beliefs, adding new religions on to existing ones; and "who are the family members" may be different for them than for us, often including extended family and close friends. By contrast, a systemic assessment often includes a genogram, a family map which the family members help the therapist draw, which shows who is in their family and support networks, and the relationships between the persons (Canda, 1989; McGoldrick & Gerson, 1985). Two or three generations are included in the genogram, which supports the Asian emphasis on ancestors. The drawing of a genogram can get the family unit involved, does not require sophisticated language skills, and enables the therapist to "see" the family structure from their point of view. Involving family members in the sessions with the identified client is useful for communication, since the children learn the new language faster and can help their elders understand.

As noted earlier, there are several schools of thought under the family systems perspective. An approach which seems especially useful for this population is the Milan Systemic approach (Boscolo et al., 1987), which incorporates ideas from other systemic schools, but puts more emphasis on meaning. These systemic thinkers call themselves consultants rather than therapists, and for them it is more a matter of philosophy than terminology. They can offer new options and views, but can not fix or cure. When working with these refugees, the terms themselves become important: "psychotherapist" to them implies mental illness which carries a stigma (Butcher et al., 1988), "counselor" may mean lawyer, and social workers are the people who offer goods and concrete services. The term "consultant" carries no stigma and connotes what actually happens–an outside expert offering new views on a family problem, but it is up to the family to utilize and act upon the ideas. While some may view this as inconsistent with a hierarchical view, it is possible and useful to have the therapist in charge of the sessions, but the families in charge of the larger issues of utilization and action.

Systemic family consultants work with the "significant systems" of the identified client; that is, they may work with any persons or institutions who are interested and significant in the life of the particular client, and do not limit themselves to the family system alone. This is especially important for these refugees, who may see extended families or friends as part of their family system. Furthermore, other agency helpers and persons indigenous to the community are involved in the process. Individual members of the family may also be seen alone; seeing all family members is not necessary in the systemic approaches. While larger and smaller system levels may be involved, the focus is kept on the family unit, as the key system linking the individual to the community.

Systemic therapy is process-oriented (Boscolo et al., 1987), rather than a set of procedures, which aids the helper to better understand the client system. Three key concepts of this school are neutrality, circularity, and hypothesizing, which are also the interventions used to help create change in the system (Boscolo et al., 1987). Hypothesizing is an assessment procedure, where the consultant engages in a research process with the family about the problem. After gathering information, a systemic hypothesis is formed which accounts for the behaviors of all of the persons in the system, and which forms the basis for an intervention. The "truth" of the hypothesis is not as important as its usefulness. Circular questioning is an interviewing technique based on the idea that the consultant conducts his or her research on the basis of feedback from the family in response to information obtained about relationships and differences (Penn, 1982). Family members are asked to comment on their beliefs about differences in degree or in perceptions with each other. Such questions as "who would be hurt most if–" or "on a scale of 1 to 10 how would you rate this problem?" or, "if everything was just the way you would like it to be how would it be." All members of the family or larger system discuss these questions, giving the interviewer a picture of this family's belief system, the meaning they attach to events, and how they want things to be. Thus, the therapist understands the situation from the family's perspective, rather than trying to fit behaviors and events into a preconceived framework, which may not be culturally sensitive and which actually blocks the therapist's understanding. Neutrality is the basic therapeutic stance of the systemic therapist. Neutrality refers to the therapist's attempts to see and understand all sides of the issues as presented by various system members, which translates into non-induction into the system. When there are sticky coalitions escalating against each other, this multi-positional view helps the therapist move in between the conflicting sets.

Rather than saying that the system creates the problem, these theorists view the problem as creating the system. Thus, blaming the individual, the family, or the society is not seen as useful, but the existing situation is viewed as a creation of the family's attempt to solve a problem. The intervention is not intended to give a new blue print for action but to help the system get unstuck. An intervention is often organized around helping system members view the situation differently, thus seeing new options. This may involve positive connotation of intent; for example, if the parents or school personnel view the intent behind a youth's behavior more positively, the youth may see the attempts of others to stop his behavior in a different light, too. This kind of therapy goes hand in hand with changes in the larger systems; these interventions are useful in getting the other helpers to shift their views of the family.

Since some topics are taboo for discussion with this population, the techniques of telling stories and using metaphors are helpful. This systemic framework is a therapeutic stance, under which specific techniques from many schools are utilized. It is a useful training and therapeutic model for work with refugee families, because it is an approach which is not culturally specific, but which is sensitive to the cultural context.

CASE EXAMPLE

As part of this training grant, a Vietnamese graduate student in social work, who was a refugee, was trained to use an integrated systems approach in work with Southeast Asian refugee families. Families were referred to the refugee family service training program from social agencies, and treated conjointly by the student and grant faculty. Work with one particular family is used here to illustrate the application of systemic concepts in treating refugee families and in training students to do so.

Stage 1. The student was taught this systemic approach step by step, using Papp's (1983) outline of stages. In the first stage, two things need to be accomplished: the therapist needs to ''join'' the family, and a clear and specific problem definition needs to be obtained. The student was encouraged to join the family by listening empathically to the family's view of the situation. Next, the following problem definition was elicited from the mother and the referral source: the mother was a single parent who had lost control of her oldest son who had dropped out of high school; he was not respectful to her, did not follow the rules of the home, and he was a bad example for the four younger children who looked up to him. The mother's hope was to regain some control of the children.

Stage 2. Next, the student learned to conduct a systemic assessment, looking at the problem in context. The mother had very little ability to speak English, less than anticipated, so the student and the children translated for the faculty therapist. This language barrier had served to isolate the mother, and it put the children in charge of her in many situations. The mother had just lost her job in a laundry, which had further isolated her. She was depressed at the time of the first interview, feeling that she had failed at her job and at child raising. Other contextual factors included the fact that she was not accepted by other members of the Vietnamese community in this small academic community because she had come from a lower social economic class in Vietnam, and her children were born out of wedlock by different fathers. She felt overwhelmed in this strange culture with no friends and few resources.

A genogram was drawn with the mother to assess her connections. Care had to be taken not to invade her privacy, so questions about the fathers of her children were minimal. Ages, relationships, relatives, and contact with people back home were noted. She was not close to or in contact with parents or siblings in Vietnam, but she had an adult son there whom she wanted us to help bring here. She also asked that we "straighten out" her kids and get her a job. We noted that many other helpers were involved, including the Department of Human Services, the State Employment Service, the church sponsor who had referred to us, and school counselors.

Stage 3. Next, based on the assessment, a systemic hypothesis was developed, that the son's acting out behavior served the purpose of getting more helpers involved in the family so that the mother would not be so lonely. It had worked, too; she had helpers from every service sector, and she was trying now to get us involved in the same projects. Furthermore, the son's behavior served the purpose of giving her a problem to focus on which could distract her from the larger and more overwhelming problem: her isolation and loneliness. We also hypothesized that the son's taking over the family authority was his way of respecting the culture, since he was a male emerging into adulthood at eighteen. The mother was allowing him to do so, because of the cultural norm for the male to be in charge, but this conflicted with her view that the parent should be in charge of the offspring. The generational hierarchy was further upset by the children learning the language and the culture faster than the mother, putting them in charge of many situations.

Stage 4. This systemic hypothesis was the basis for the plan of intervention. We decided not to get involved in providing direct services since so many agencies were already doing those services. We agree with Imber-Black (1988) that too much help can undermine a family's sense of competence, and in this situation that seemed to be the case. We agreed to provide short term intervention to help the mother be in charge of the family, to encourage her to continue with the other helpers for other services, and to consult with those agencies as needed. She was encouraged to attend English as a Second Language classes and the social activities in her low rent apartment complex. Most of the renters there were not Vietnamese, which was useful because she did not want to socialize with Vietnamese, but she needed language skills to socialize with others.

While the mother was seen alone once, the main intervention was to involve all family members in the sessions, and to get the son to utilize his authority with the younger children by putting him in charge of enforcing the mother's rules and being her helper. This gave the family a much needed hierarchical structure; the mother was put in charge of the family, but the eldest son was second in command. The mother now had an ally, and the son's self esteem was improved as the label was changed from bad boy to responsible man. Further, the Job Corps got him into a training program, which removed him from the home for a period of time, allowing the mother to regain some authority before the new structure was put into effect. A plan was worked out with the younger children where they would help the mother in small ways around the house, and an Asian (but not Vietnamese) male graduate student was found to tutor the children in their English and other studies and to serve as a role model for them. It was hoped that his positive influence on the younger children could counteract some of the messages the older son had given them about what it is like to grow up in America; he had been involved with the negative side of teen age life.

Stage 5. The family therapy was terminated after three months, during which the sessions had gradually decreased in frequency. The tutor stayed on for two more months, and the mother telephoned the Vietnamese graduate student on occasion. There were still problems, and they will continue, but the goals of restructuring the hierarchy and reframing the problem were met. From a systemic view, we perturbed the system and created structural change with the belief that small changes ripple through the system and result in continuous change. It is hoped that this minimal intervention will help them to utilize the other helpers more effectively.

Our methods of intervention were minimalist by design. It can be argued that many deeper problems, both at the individual and societal level, were untouched. While this may be true, we believe that too much intervention at the psychological level is often harmful for persons already coping with rapid change. The main needs of these families are for concrete services at first, and these needs are usually met by other agencies. In the situations referred to us, we found it most useful to serve as consultants to those agencies and to intervene therapeutically only around an immediate problem.

DISCUSSION

In this paper, a training project for work with Southeast Asian refugees using an integrated family system's approach, developed by this author for this project, is described and discussed and its usefulness argued. There are many approaches which fall under the rubric of family systems, and in our project we used a model integrating structural, strategic, life cycle, and Milan systemic therapies. We found this model useful at all three levels of our project work: consulting with agencies serving this population, training students for this work, and intervening clinically with the refugees themselves. The particular case example used here was chosen because it demonstrates how these systemic therapies were integrated into a unified treatment plan and taught to a student.

In this case situation, contextual and life cycle factors (Carter & McGoldrick, 1988) were taken into account, which is especially important for refugee families. The focus on minimal intervention aimed at interrupting a problem sequence was borrowed from the strategic school (Haley, 1976), while the reframing and restructuring hierarchies were structural techniques (Minuchin, 1974) which were consistent with their culture. Basing the intervention on a systemic hypothesis was drawn from the Milan theorists (Boscolo et al., 1987). All of the systems approaches are short term, problem-focused, and de-emphasize pathology. We found these properties of systemic theory to be useful with refugee families because they are respectful of privacy, they do not try to change too much too fast, and they allow for a wide range of interventive tools from which specific case plans can be designed.

We found these concepts to be useful in training and consulting, also, because the sessions with the trainees are organized around developing a hypothesis and planning an intervention. Information is gathered around the presenting problem, and stages of intervention are clearly identified. Papp's (1983) book was useful in this training because it presents assessment and treatment in a step by step approach.

In summary, we found this integrated family systems model useful in our work with Southeast Asian refugee families and in training others to do so. Although there is no longer a funded demonstrated project, several of us who were involved in this project continue to explore ways to serve this population. It is hoped that this paper will generate further interest in examining ways in which systemic therapies can be integrated and used for this purpose.

REFERENCES

Ben-Porath, Y. (1987). Issues in the psycho-social adjustment of refugees. NIMH Contract No. 278-85-0024 (CH), Refugee Assistance Program–Mental Health: Technical Assistance Center. Minneapolis, MN: University of Minnesota.

Boscolo, L., Cecchin, G., Hoffman, L., & Penn, P. (1987). *Milan systemic family therapy*. New York: Basic Books.

Butcher, J., Egli, E., Shiota, N., & Ben-Porath, Y. (1988). Psychological interventions with refugees. NIMH Contract No. 278-85-0024 (CH), Refugee Assistance Program–Mental Health: Technical Assistance Center. Minneapolis, MN: University of Minnesota.

Canda, E. (1989). Therapeutic use of writing and other media with Southeast Asian refugees. *Journal of Independent Social Work, 4,* 2, 47-60.

Carter, B. & McGoldrick, M. (1988). *The changing family life cycle: A framework for family therapy*. New York: Gardner Press.

Charron, D., & Ness, R. (1981). Emotional distress among Vietnamese adolescents. *Journal of Refugee Resettlement, 3* (May), 7-15.

Deinard, A. (1988). Models of professional and paraprofessional training in refugee mental health, task VI training. NIMH Contract #278-65-0024 (CH), Refugee Assistance Program–Mental Health: Technical Assistance Center. Minneapolis, MN: University of Minnesota.

Friedman, J., Tobin, J., & Koschmann, N. (1981). Working with refugees: A manual for paraprofessionals, volume III: Intercultural counseling and interviewing skills. Chicago, IL: Refugee Resettlement Service.

Haley, J. (1976). *Problem solving therapy*. San Francisco: Jossey-Bass.

Hirayama, H. & Cetingok, M. (1988). Empowerment: a social work approach for Asian immigrants. *Social Casework*, 69, 1, 41-47.

Ho, M.K. (1987). *Family therapy with ethnic minorities*. Newbury Park, CA: Sage Publications.

Hoshino, G., Bamford, P., & DuBois, D. (1987). Culturally sensitive refugee mental health training programs. NIMH Contract 278-85-0024 (CH), Refugee Assistance Program–Mental Health: Technical Assistance Center. Minneapolis, MN: University of Minnesota.

Imber-Black, E. (1988). *Families and larger systems*. New York: The Guilford Press.

Jaranson, J., & Bamford, P. (1987). Program models for mental health treatment of refugees. NIMH Contract No. 278-85-0024 (CH), Refugee Assistance Program–Mental Health: Technical Assistance Center. Minneapolis, MN: University of Minnesota.

Keeney, B.P. & Ross J.M. (1985). *Mind in therapy: Constructing systemic family therapies*. New York: Basic Books.

McGoldrick, M., & Gerson, R. (1985). *Genograms in family assessment*. New York: W.W. Norton & Co.

Minuchin, S. (1974). *Families and family therapy*. Cambridge, MA: Harvard University Press.

Murphy, G., & Frey, L. (1988). *Casebook and training guide in Southeast Asian refugee mental health*. Boston, MA: Boston University School of Social Work.

Papp, P. (1983). *The process of change*. New York: Guilford Press.

Penn, P. (1982). Circular questioning. *Family Process*, 21, 3, 267-280.

Team Associates, (Eds.). (1980). Social/cultural customs: Similarities and differences between Vietnamese, Cambodians, Hmong, and Lao. Washington DC: US Department of Labor, Contract No. 99-7-998-36-17.

U.S. Department of State, Bureau of Refugee Programs, (March 31, 1988). Summary of Refugee Admissions, Fiscal Year 1988: Author.

Westermeyer, J. (1986). Models of assessment, treatment, and prevention for social adjustment and mental health of refugees. Technical Assistance Center. Minneapolis, MN: University of Minnesota.

The Indochinese Refugees:
A Perspective
from Various Stress Theories

Diane Bernier

SUMMARY. Cambodian, Laotian and Vietnamese refugees who have come to North American host countries via the South Asian camps have been exposed to many potentially traumatic events and have been submitted to an alienating migration process. A comprehensive analysis of their experience both in refugee camps and North American host countries is facilitated by the use of various stress theories. The stressors of change, acculturation, bereavement and trauma are identified with regard to the migration process of the Indochinese refugees as well as to the pre- and post-migration period. Some implications for practice in social, physical and mental health settings are underlined: in particular a sensitivity to the meaning of physical illness within this population, to the cultural reticence towards mental health consultation, to the possibility of longterm vulnerability to post-traumatic stress disorders and to increasing value conflicts within the family. Intervention experiences both in the South Asian refugee camps and in North American host countries suggests the importance of traditional healers and natural support networks.

The difficulties of immigrants and the plight of refugees have received much attention. However, the migration process of some groups of refugees is marked by a particular experience: that of the

Diane Bernier, MSW, is Associate Professor at the School of Social Work, University of Montreal, P.O.B. 6128, Branch A, Montreal (Quebec) Canada H3C 3J7.

This paper was presented at the XXV International Congress of Schools of Social Work, Lima, 1990.

15

temporary stay in a refugee camp. This is a foreign reality for many North American workers currently employed in health and social agencies to which former refugee camp residents address themselves or are being referred for service. With this in mind, and building on previous stress-related research (Bernier & Gaston, 1989), the author undertook an informal study of the stressful conditions of the refugee camps in Thaïland.

When thinking of refugee camps, one expects to observe cramped living quarters, food shortages or restrictions, limited water supplies and primitive hygiene facilities. All of these exist in South Asian refugee camps, but also many other realities, such as cultural differences between refugee groups and consequent friction, massive powerlessness related to refugee status, lengthy duration of stay for so many residents, along with the traumatic quality of prior events and of the arrival at camp. These observations of camp life and its consequences on subsequent experiences in the North American host countries, will be analyzed within the context of various stress theories familiar to the investigator. In subsequent considerations about the implications of these theories for practice, reference will be made to intervention experiences observed in the South Asian camps and reported in the main North American host countries.

STRESS RELATED TO ACCULTURATION

In the Thaï refugee camps, residents of various nationalities are grouped in different geographical locations. This has been done to minimize friction stemming from past political history. The use of the generic appellation (Indochese) when referring to the Laotians, Cambodians and Vietnamese can be misleading. Although they have much in common (geographic proximity, long-standing civilizations, the relatively recent experience of living decades under French protectorate rules and then acceding to independence, war and political turmoil over the last fifty years), they have different histories, languages, religions and cultures. Cohabitation has proven to be difficult.

The cultural differences between residents and some camp staff have on occasion been an additional source of difficulties, as is illustrated in the following incident. An epidemic had occurred in the camps and medical authorities proceeded with a relevant vaccination program for the residents. A sub-group of tribal origins, resisting the procedure hid when called, and avoided vaccination in a variety of ways. For members of this group, "contagion" was an inconceivable reality since sickness, in their culture, comes from the spirits. Medical authorities had to resort to temporary quarantine in order to go ahead with the protective measures.

However the stress due to cultural factors is even more prevalent once the refugees arrive in the North American host countries. Here they will share, with various types of migrants, the experience of acculturation. This phenomenon has been described by Bhagat (1985) as

> a process of accommodation and adaptation, on the part of members of a minority or ethnic culture, to the dominant cultural values of a majority culture. (p. 327)

Trying to define culture in this context, Jacob (1987) quotes Simon (1975) as follows:

> Culture, in its ethnographic sense, is the complex ensemble of knowledge, beliefs, art, morals, law, customs along with all aptitudes and habits acquired by man as member of a society.[1] (p. 67)

Changes in these various elements are viewed as stressors, i.e., sources of strain, possibly leading to psychosomatic symptoms, along with feelings of alienation, marginalization and identity confusion (Berry et al., 1987). According to Hopkins-Kavanagh and Sananikone (1981), researchers agree that the stress or strain experienced by immigrants is more intense when the "distance" between the immigrant's culture and that of the majority group is larger. In the case of the Indochinese refugee, the cultural distance is a substantial one. Indeed, not only is the spoken language different but also the written. With regard to religion, Buddhism, Taoism and Confucianism are very distant from the various forms of Christianity that prevail in North America. Dance and music, to mention only two forms of artistic activity, belong to completely different traditions. Food and eating habits are equally divergent from those prevalent in the host countries. Among family customs, the importance of the extended family and of paternal authority are a far cry from our nuclear family and our concept of children's rights. Last, their valuing of emotional control (i.e., inhibition) and their views on mental health are opposed to the beliefs of countries where, for instance, the primal scream, Gestalt therapy and bioenergetics have flourished. Differences in values also aggravate the generational conflicts between parents and their offspring and this will become a source of problems long after re-settlement.

The material aspects of a culture are not to be neglected in these considerations: objects and places. In this regard, these refugees, often from an underdeveloped region, find themselves in an environment where an elaborate technology is commonplace: microwave cooking, electrical appliances, computer-banking, etc. Peasants (for instance many of the Laotian refugees) must live in an urban context, quite removed from nature, in high-rise dwellings. Finally the change in climate, particularly in Canada, contributes to additional cultural changes in habit and life style.

Many authors, including Fox (1984), Hopkins-Kavanagh and Sananikone (1981), and Chan and Lam (1983) do not hesitate to use the term "culture shock."

STRESS RELATED TO BEREAVEMENT

Physical constraints are numerous in refugee camps leading to overcrowding, lack of water, imposed food and related loss of vital space, intimacy and freedom of movement. But no less important is the loss of power that is inherent in the status of refugee. In some camps (e.g., Panet Nikhom) newcomers having no identity papers are jailed until identity can be established (a process which can take several months). The lack of equipment and staff gives rise to regrettable incidents, such as that involving a young mother of three children who came to the attention of camp authorities six years after her arrival. Once they are admitted, the residents are totally dependent on administrative processes over which they have no control. Scarcity of resources and staff, along with the importance of bureaucratic procedures contributes to the alienating aspects of this humanitarian endeavor. This alienation is coupled in many instances with general idleness. Poverty, idleness, and alienation contribute to substantial losses in self-esteem.

In addition, the refugee does not choose a host country; he waits to be chosen. He can only hope that the camp authorities will choose to present him to the selection committees of various countries. There are thousands with the same expectation . . . The host countries have eligibility criteria that are sometimes arbitrary, for example a nuclear family will be turned down because of an accompanying sister-in-law; some countries will not accept young unattached persons, etc. Mental health, language proficiency and employability are important choice factors over which the camp residents have little immediate power. The passive waiting goes on even after acceptance by a host country, since the date of departure from camp is sometimes only known several months later. For instance, in 1988, this waiting period lasted approximately 11 months before actual entry into Canada.[2]

Intense reactions to losses are observed in the months preceding departure from refugee camps. A mental health consultant in the transit camp of Panet Nikhom reported major crises and suicidal attempts during this period when the various losses become more concrete and more definitive.[3]

Although bereavement is not usually presented within the framework of stress, it nevertheless occupies a very legitimate place in this conceptual arena. Henry and Meehan (1981) in their psychophysiological model of stress, refer to bereavement as a stressor associated with a neuro-hormonal reaction of the hypophyso-adrenal axis: it is considered as distress. In this perspective, distress, such as for instance, bereavement, helplessness and loss of control are associated with the production of the ACTH hormone and conducive to mental and physical illness; distress is to be distinguished from effort and tension (involved in what some authors call positive stress) which is simply associated with the production of adrenalin. Other authors have mentioned the importance of this fundamental distinction between effort and distress or action inhibition (Laborit, 1979; Frankenhauser, 1986).

Once they have arrived in North America, these refugees must resume "normal" living without their belongings or their cherished mementos. In addition, they suffer further cultural and relational losses. Brown (1982) insists on the emotional impact of these multiple losses. In an exploratory study of Indochinese refugees having attempted suicide, Curtis (1982) describes reactive depression and separation from loved ones as the best indicators of life-threatening behaviors.

An interesting study was conducted by Chan and Lam (1983); it included an analysis of dream content in a sample of Vietnamese refugees living in Montreal.

> . . . dream contents (. . .) reveal a predominant and overwhelming preoccupation with the past. (p. 8)

In the opinion of these authors, the feeling of loss in their subjects is comparable to that of bereavement. Many of these refugees experience chronic anxiety related to the loss of loved ones or the lack of information concerning their fate. In these subjects, dreams are repetitive, recurrent and always take place in a Vietnamese setting. This feeling of loss constitutes, according to the authors, a primary mental preoccupation which consumes much time and energy. This attachment to the past has been described by other authors: Zwingmann (1973) developed the concept of "nostalgic fixation," to which he adds an idealization of the past.

These refugees therefore must accomplish an important "working through" of grief before they can enjoy, once more, gratifying objects and activities.

STRESS RELATED TO CHANGE

According to the testimony of various professionals, the average length of stay in the camp is two years.[4] Refugees with close relatives (such as a spouse) in a host country stand a chance of moving on more quickly, but for the others it means that camp life will go on for several years. This will therefore lead to substantial changes in life style and living conditions.

Selye (1956) initiated the interest in stress associated with adaptational efforts. Change is one instance that requires such efforts. Within this framework, Holmes and Rahe (1967) pursued an interest in change-related "life events": they developed the Social Readjustment Rating Scale, based on a list of events that are experienced over the years by most adults (death of a loved one, addition of a family member, marriage, change at work, indebtedness, move to another residence, etc.). This instrument has been used to study the relationship between the rate of change and the onset of illness. Although this correlation is often weak (from .12 to .30, according to Folkman and Lazarus, 1985, p. 310) and fraught with methodological difficulties (Amiel-Lebigre, 1986; Nadeau, 1989) the interest for this question of illness susceptibility has led to a number of studies (Dohrenwend and Dohrenwend, 1974; Thoits, 1983).

This theme has given rise to controversy. Some authors state that the quantity of change is sufficient to favor the appearance of psychological problems, others believe that only undesirable events lead to psychological difficulties. The goal of this study is not to settle this controversy, since the refugees under study in this paper experience both types of change. As victims of socio-political events and objects of international benevolence, the camp refugees experience much undesired change associated with unpleasant or painful consequences. Further sections will deal with these aspects. At this point, the quantity of changes associated with their particular type of migration will be emphasized.

First, the change in the social environment that prompts a person to flee in spite of major risks, must be important and multi-dimensional: it threatens survival. In addition, refugees who go through the refugee camps experience a fairly long migration process. A second wave of substantial change in living conditions is thus experienced, associated with a loss of freedom. The hardships of camp life are, in the opinion of this investigator, largely underestimated. Finally, in the post-migration phase, another series of changes will affect status, everyday life and habits and will trigger more "life events."

Building on previous transcultural research involving the Social Readjustment Scale, Masuda, Lin and Tazuma (1980) used this instrument for a study of migration and post-migration changes in a group of Vietnamese refugees of the first wave (1975-76). They observed a substantial rise (four times more) in the change ratings over this two year period. In the second year (which was the first year of post-migration) some scores dropped (i.e., personal change), some maintained a high level (i.e., life style, finances), while others rose (i.e., work, spouse, difficulties with the law and learning institutions). Several items causing this increase in the score were work related: change in financial status, readjustment in business, difficulties with the boss, change in working conditions, change in type of work, the spouse starting or stopping work. These authors (Lin, Tazuma, Masuda, 1979) observed a high rate of unemployment (46%) and professional disqualification (18%) of persons having had a prestigious occupation in Vietnam and estimated that the menial jobs held by the newly arrived would not be rewarding or conducive to heightened self-esteem.

Other studies have emphasized the importance of work-related changes. In a comparative study of Vietnamese refugees of the first wave and those (the boat people) who arrived later via the camps, Nguyen and Henkin (1982) reported twice as much difficulty in finding a well-paid job. The same difficulties with employment have been observed for Laotians (Hopkins-Kavanagh and Sananikone, 1981); the loss of prestige and of subsequent self-esteem has been emphasized. Professional disqualification is a painful experience, particularly if it is seen as a long-lasting one, equally painful are work-related discrimination and daily harassment.[5] The loss of prestige felt by the male becomes even more painful if his wife enters the labor market. Citing a number of authors, the Canadian Task Force on Mental Health Issues Affecting Immigrants and Refugees (1988) is of the opinion that employment status has more impact on the psychological well being of migrants than pre-migration stress or separation from the family. Although this might not apply to specific groups of refugees, it does point to the centrality of work in the adaptation process and to the stress related to changes in this area.

All these elements favour the recognition of the magnitude of change-related stressors that South Asian refugees must cope with.

STRESS RELATED TO TRAUMA

Threat to survival is the essence of trauma. For many Indochinese refugees, having experienced war, famine, persecution, and forced labour, being in a refugee camp may not appear as a traumatic event. However camp experience is a changing phenomenon. Geographic location and population input have changed over the years. Some instances, as described by staff having a long-standing camp experience, may have been traumatic for some individuals. Refugees have been known to arrive by waves, sometimes in very large numbers, contributing to overcrowding in unsuitable facilities; such as an island without water, or shelters where residents must sleep in turns, for lack of space to lie down.

One of the particular aspects of trauma is its capacity to be a source of distress over very long periods. Associated disorders can be intense and immediate, but may also be delayed (and occur several years later) or chronic (i.e., never to be overcome). Post-traumatic stress theory has been very helpful in drawing attention to the duration of vulnerability in victims of trauma. The most frequently observed symptoms are intense mental phenomena: repeated nightmares, avoidance behaviours, sudden aggressive fits, dissociative phenomena.

The psychiatric definition of trauma (DSM III) refers to an event which is outside usual human experience and is accompanied by emotional distress. Kolb (1988) draws particular attention to the emotional component which, in his opinion, is the critical etiological factor: intensity, repetition and duration of a fear from which there is no immediate escape. This emotion reaches levels of helpless terror and despair. In addition, Benyakar (1989) highlights the destructuring aspect of the phenomena and the accompanying loss of autonomy: catastrophic threat and chaotic response.

The pre-migration history of Indochinese refugees is fraught with potentially traumatic events: war against invaders, genocide, persecution, labor camps, flight through the jungle, boat or raft journey on a dangerous sea infested with pirates (as documented by Landgren, 1989), repeated rapes. In a study of a group of Laotian refugees, Nicassio and his collaborators (1986) tried to identify the relative importance of emigration stress, acculturative stress and degree of proficiency in the language of the host country, in the onset of depression. They concluded that emigration stress and the absence of language proficiency were the best predictors of depression in their subjects.

Possible prolonged vulnerability at the mental health level has thus been identified for this target group of refugees.

PRACTICE APPLICATIONS

The proposed stress theories have implications for the helping process.

Culture

One might think that acculturative stress tends to diminish as time of residence in the host country passes.

It is only over time, with repeated failures and frustrations, that the psychological stresses of acculturation accumulate. (Dressler and Bernal, 1982, p. 34)

In addition, value conflicts that arise in bringing up children in the host countries usually become more severe as children grow older. These long-term effects related to these aspects of refugee experience should be known to staff working in various agencies, particularly in non-ethnic organizations.

In addition, the cultural resistance to mental health consultation in "Western" settings is a very deepset one. The traditional importance of "saving face" leads families to try and solve problems within the family without external consultation. The expression of emotions is not part of their tradition (Lee, 1989; Fox, 1984). In addition, their conception of mental illness differs considerably from the Western concept. The Indochinese see it as the result of an energetic disequilibrium and the possession by evil spirits. Rites of purification with lustral waters and exorcism prevail in the traditional healing of mental health problems.

A recourse to traditional doctors and healers, when possible, is an efficient treatment in many cases. Experiences of this type were observed in the refugee camps of Thaïland: Hiegel (1984) has been influential in setting up the Center for Traditional Medicine where Kmer doctors treat both mental and physical disorders; Western professionals rarely see patients, rather they provide support to the medical and voluntary staff of traditional orientation. This receptiveness on the part of Western medical staff is not generally evidenced in the North American literature. Among the exceptions is a case study reported by Tobin and Friedman (1983) in Chicago, illustrating the benefits of an exorcism practiced by a shaman on a twenty-two year old Hmong suffering from panic attacks. The limits on interventions of a traditional type are reached in mental illnesses of a psychotic nature (one camp had a small psychiatric unit). Considering cultural differences, Western therapists have come to the conclusion that treatments that are brief, active and focused on action are more helpful than those that are long-term and centered on psychological content.

Bereavement

The previous analysis of the emotional impact of multiple losses and subsequent grief leads to considerations about the importance of social support. The Indochinese belong to a culture where the extended family and the neighborhood are of utmost importance; their uprooting is therefore particularly painful. Interventions must take this reality into account in order to be relevant. Tung (1986) mentions, for instance, the importance of involving the family in treatment and giving preference to home visits.

Within this perspective, a project from the School of Social Work of Fordham University (New York) is worth mentioning (Fox, 1984). Conscious of the hostility of the social environment, the project directors decided on a ''community'' approach to service the Indochinese refugees. Working from accessible premises in the neighborhood, social workers aimed at identifying, stimulating and reinforcing the natural support network. Priority was given to home visits, mutual help groups and interest groups together with community education about existing services and citizen rights. The authors concluded that these services, in addition to the training provided to volunteers and social workers were the most efficient components of the overall project. Trying to alter existing services and make them more relevant does not appear to be the most urgent priority, particularly in communities character-ized by recently arrived refugees.

Change

The theory on stress associated with "life events" gives particu-lar meaning to the onset of illness; in this perspective, the latter appears as a symptom of adaptational difficulties related to change. Medical consultation is the only one that Indochinese refugees use spontaneously, both in camps and in host countries. Their utiliza-tion of social and psychiatric services is very limited (Kinzie, 1988).

A strong association between problems of physical and mental health has been evidenced by Lin, Tazuma and Masuda (1979). In their sample of Vietnamese refugees, half the subjects consulting for physical complaints had emotional problems as measured by mental health tests. As noted by Lee (1989), several authors have mentioned the prevalence of somatization in this group of refugees. Medical consultation becomes a strategic opportunity for early diagnosis of psychosocial and mental health problems. Staff in medical settings should be fully aware of the possible implications of physical illness particularly in this group of refugees.

Trauma

As a working knowledge of post-traumatic stress disorder be-comes more widespread, diagnostic errors bearing undesirable social consequences (i.e., unwarranted child placements and psychi-atric hospitalizations) will become less frequent. Kinzie (1989) and Westermeyer (1983) explain diagnostic errors by the fact that post-traumatic symptoms appear many years later and that mental health experts who are not fully aware of these problems carry out incom-plete investigations.

Westermeyer (1989) has described at length the specificity of diagnosis, treatment, prevention and research in a transcultural perspective. Finally, Lee and Lu (1989) have focused on particular-ities of such treatment for Indochinese refugees. In the opinion of several authors (Kinzie, 1989; Westermeyer, 1983; Lee and Lu, 1989), Cambodians and Laotians are groups among which the incidence and severity of mental health problems are worth noting.

CONCLUSION

The goal of this paper is to make mental health and welfare workers fully aware of the numerous difficulties that South Asian refugees have faced in the course of their migration process. The use of several stress theories seemed a good way to construct an overall vision of this type of refugee experience. In doing so, much importance has been given to stressors that impact physical and mental health. The latter, in the opinion of the author, constitutes for these refugees major obstacles to learning and creativity which are such crucial elements in an adaptational context. The learning of language, working skills and other abilities requires receptivity and energy rather than physical or emotional pain. Without these skills, the poverty and alienation of these refugees may become chronic.

Work with this type of client requires specific training. In the author's experience, anthropology and history have much to contribute in the understanding of Indochinese refugees. Elements from these disciplines should be part of the prerequisite knowledge for this type of work. In addition, substantial insights into depression and post-traumatic syndrome should be part of the knowledge base for staff. Furthermore, mediation and community work skills should be central elements in training for practice. Respect for another culture leads to treating the other person as an equal. Thus, mediation is a good framework for this type of intervention. The importance of the network in Indochinese culture justifies the need for specific skills in community work. Knowledge, patience and receptivity are key elements for successful work with these clients.

Some of the observations in this study apply to other refugees. The analysis has pointed out several key factors such as the duration of the migration process, the stay in a refugee camp, cultural distance, traumatic experiences (forced labor camps and torture being the most difficult to overcome) and the importance of relational and material losses.

NOTES

1. Translation by the author.
2. As reported to the author by camp workers, June 1988.
3. Personal communication to the author, June 1988.
4. As reported to the author by professionals working in the transit camp of Panet Nikhom, June 1988.
5. As reported by Mr. Chan, Cambodian refugee, in his presentation at the Annual Meeting of the Canadian Mental Health Association (Montreal section), May 5th, 1990.

REFERENCES

Amiel-Lebigre, F. (1986). Méthodes d'évaluation des événements stressants de la vie. *Encyclopédie médico-chirurgicale*, Psychiatrie, 37401E10, 11-1988, 4 p.

Benyakar, M., Kutz, I., Dasberg, H. and Stern, M. (1989). The collapse of a structure: A structural approach to trauma. *Journal of Traumatic Stress, 2*, (4), 431-449.

Bernier, D. and Gaston, L. (1989). Differential efficacy of educational and somatic stress management programs across two samples. *Canadian Journal of Program Evaluation, 1.*

Bhagat, R.S. (1985). The Role of stressful life events in organizational behavior and human performance. In T.A. Beehr and R.S. Bhagat, (Eds.), *Human Stress and Cognition in Organizations: An Integrated Perspective.* New York: John Wiley & Sons.

Brown, G. (1982). Issues in the resettlement of Indochinese refugees. *Social Casework, 63*, (3), 155-159.

Chan, K.B. and Lam, L. (1983). Resettlement of Vietnamese-Chinese refugees in Montreal, Canada: some socio-psychological problems and dilemmas. *Canadian Ethnic Studies, 15*, (1), 1-17.

Curtis Alley, J. (1982). Life-threatening indicators among the Indochinese refugees. *Suicide and Life-Threatening Behavior, 12*, (1), 46-52.

Dohrenwend, B.S. and Dohrenwend, B.P. (Eds.) (1974). *Stressful Life Events: their Nature and Effects.* New York: Wiley.

Dressler, W., Bernal, H. (1982). Acculturation and stress in a low income puerto rican community. *Journal of Human Stress, 8*, (3), 32-38.

Folkman, S. et Lazarus, R. (1985). *Stress, appraisal and coping.* New York: Springer.

Fox, R. (1984). The Indochinese: Strategies for health survival. *International Journal of Social Psychiatry, 30*, (1&2), 287-291.

Frankenhauser, M. (1986). A psychobiological framework for research on human stress and coping. In M. A Appley and R. Trumbull (Eds.), *Dynamics of*

Stress: Physiological, psychological and social perspectives. New York: Plenum Press.

Henry, J.P. and Meehan, J.P. (1981). Psychosocial stimuli, physiological specificity and cardiovascular disease. In H. Weine, M.A. Hofer and A.J. Stunkard (Eds.), *Brain, Behavior and Bodily Disease* (pp. 305-333). New York: Raven Press.

Hiegel, J.P. (1984). Collaboration with traditional healers: Experience in refugees' mental care. *International Journal of Mental Health, 12,* (3), 30-43.

Holmes, T.H. and Rahe, R.H. (1967). The Social readjustment rating scale. *Journal of Psychosomatic Research, 11,* 213-218.

Hopkins-Kavanagh, K. and Sananikone, P. (1981). Migration, mental health and the Laotian refugee. *Migration News,* (1), 15-23.

Jacob, A. (1987). Modèles d'intervention et communautés ethno-culturelles: entre l'imaginaire et le réel. *Apprentissage et socialisation, 10,* (2), 99-106.

Kinzie, J.D. (1988). The psychiatric effects of massive trauma on Cambodian refugees. In J.P. Wilson, Z. Harel and B. Kahana (eds.), *Human Adaptation to Extreme Stress.* New York: Plenum.

Kinzie, J.D. (1989). Therapeutic approaches to traumatized Cambodian refugees. *Journal of Traumatic Stress, 2,* (1), 75-92.

Kinzie, J.D. and Boehnlein, J.K. (1989). Post-traumatic psychosis among Cambodian refugees. *Journal of Traumatic Stress, 2,* (2), 185-198.

Kolb, L.C. (1988). A critical survey of hypotheses regarding post-traumatic stress disorders in light of recent research findings. *Journal of Traumatic Stress, 1,* (3), 291-304.

Laborit, H. (1979). *L'inhibition de l'action.* Paris, Montréal: Masson.

Landgren, K. (1989). Ceux qui ont eu de la chance. *Réfugiés,* 27-28.

Lee, E. and Lu, F. (1989). Assessment and treatment of Asian-American survivors of Mass violence. *Journal of Traumatic Stress, 2,* (1), 93-120.

Lin, K.M., Tazuma, L., Masuda, M. (1979). Adaptational problems of Vietnamese refugees. 1. Health and mental health status. *Archives of General Psychiatry,* (36), 955-961.

Masuda, M., Lin, K., Tazuma, L. (1980). Adaptation problems of Vietnamese refugees: II. Life changes and perception of life events. *Archives of General Psychiatry, 37,* 447-450.

Nadeau, L. (1989). La mesure des événements et des difficultés de vie: un cas particulier des problèmes méthodologiques liés à l'étude de l'étiologie sociale des troubles mentaux. *Santé mentale au Québec, 14,* (1), 121-131.

Nguyen, L.T. and Henkin, A.B. (1982). Vietnamese refugees in the United States: Adaptation and transitional status. *The Journal of Ethnic Studies, 9,* (4), 101-116.

Nicassio, P.M., Solomon, G.S., Guest, S.S., McCullough, B.S. (1986). Emigration stress and language proficiency as correlates of depression in a sample of Southeast Asian refugees. *International Journal of Social Psychiatry, 32,* (1), 23-28.

Report of the Canadian Task Force on Mental Health Issues Affecting Immigrants and Refugees (1988). *Review of the literature on migrant mental health.*

Selye, H. (1956). *The Stress of Life.* New York: McGraw-Hill.

Thoits, P.A. (1983). Dimensions of life events as influences upon the genesis of psychological distress and associated conditions: An evaluation and synthesis of the literature. In H.B. Kaplan (Ed.), *Psychological Stress: Trends in Theory and Research.* New York: Academic Press.

Tobin, J.J. and Friedman, J. (1983). Spirits-shamans and nightmare death: Survivor stress in a Hmong refugee. *American Journal of Orthopsychiatry, 53,* (3), 439-448.

Tung, P. (1986). Les problèmes de santé mentale des Vietnamiens à Calgary: Aspects principaux et conséquences pour les services touchés. *Santé mentale au Canada,* 6-11.

Westermeyer, J. (1989). Cross-cultural care for PTSD: research, training and service needs for the future. *Journal of Traumatic Stress, 2,* (4) 515-536.

Westermeyer, J., Vang, T.F., Neider, J. (1983). Migration and mental health among Hmong refugees. Association of pre- and post-migration factors with self-rating scales. *Journal of Nervous Mental Disease, 171,* (2), 92-96.

Zwingmann, C. (1973). The nostalgic phenomenon and its exploitation. In C. Zwingmann and M. Pfister-Ammende (Eds.), *Uprooting and After.* New York: Springer-Verlag.

Refugee and Immigrant Social Service Delivery: Critical Management Issues

Cora Le-Doux
King S. Stephens

SUMMARY. Much concern has been expressed regarding the potential burden on the states to provide health, education, social and mental health services to refugees, immigrants, and newly legalized aliens. Management of social services for refugees and immigrants is an area which has not received much attention in the social work literature. Within the framework of two components of the current immigration policy, this article will examine funding, staffing, service delivery, and information system needs as critical management issues in the resettlement of refugees and in the delivery of social services to eligible legalized aliens in the United States.

INTRODUCTION

Management of social services for refugees and immigrants is an area which has not received much attention in the social work literature. The literature on these populations focuses primarily on micro level issues related to culturally appropriate treatment approaches and barriers to social service delivery. This paper will examine critical management issues in the resettlement of refugees and the delivery of social services to eligible legalized aliens in the United States such as funding, staffing, service delivery, and information system needs.

Cora Le-Doux, MSSW, CSW and King S. Stephens, MSSW, CSW-ACP, are affiliated with the School of Social Work at the University of Texas at Austin.

Immigration, voluntary and involuntary, can be viewed as either a domestic or foreign policy issue. As a domestic policy issue in the United States, immigration has been dealt with primarily through legislation and there are essentially two forms: legal (documented) and illegal (undocumented) immigration.

The terms refugee, immigrant, entrant, eligible legalized aliens, and non-immigrant are *legal* terms used by the Immigration and Naturalization Service to identify and describe individuals legally admitted to the United States. Each of these terms has its own eligibility definitions based on United States Department of Justice criteria. However, the boundaries of these categories are relative. For example, AmerAsians from Viet Nam may be categorized as either refugees or immigrants, and members of the same household/family often may have different legal statuses. For the purposes of this paper, the term refugee will be used to denote individuals eligible for social services under Office of Refugee Resettlement, Family Support Administration, of the United States Department of Health and Human Services. The term eligible legalized alien will be used to refer to individuals who adjusted their status from undocumented to documented under the amnesty provisions of the 1986 Immigration Reform and Control Act.

At the macro level, there are five basic strategies used in addressing displaced populations:

1. restrictive or exclusive legislation,
2. deportation or repatriation,
3. incarceration,
4. provision of interventions to source countries, and
5. resettlement.

Although the United States prefers to provide interventions to source countries, it has a long history as a major participant in international resettlement activities.

In the area of U.S. immigration, it is important to recognize that there are severe conflicts between strongly held sets of values. Attitudes toward immigration policy can be conceptualized along a continuum. One extreme is closed-door policy—the other end of the continuum is unrestricted, open-door policy. Political, economic, social, cultural, and historical factors; and technological advancements contribute to the tightening or relaxation of U.S. immigration policy. An effective and clear-cut policy of exclusion (closed-door), or wide-open border (open-door), would mobilize a strong reaction not only from opponents, but from relatively uninvolved persons and groups. This makes it difficult to adopt "rational" immigration policies.

The bulk of federal government services to refugees and eligible legalized aliens is provided within the framework of these two programs: the Refugee Resettlement Program and the State Legalization Impact Assistance Grants. These two components of current immigration policy will provide the framework for a discussion about management of social service delivery to refugees and eligible legalized aliens and are described below.

PERTINENT POLICY COMPONENTS

A comprehensive historical overview of U.S. immigration policy is beyond the scope of this article. However, there are two components of the current policy which must be addressed, and provide the framework for a discussion of management issues in social service provision to refugees and eligible legalized aliens: (1) the Office of Refugee Resettlement Program; and (2) the State Legalization Impact Assistance Grants.

The Refugee Resettlement Program (RRP) is under the auspices of the Office of Refugee Resettlement (ORR), Family Support Administration (FSA) of the U.S. Department of Health and Human Services (HHS). Funds for refugee reception and resettlement services are made available to HHS by the Department of State on an annual basis. These funds are allocated in accordance with refugee admissions numbers determined by the President, in consultation with Congress. The funding is channeled from the ORR to the states. The states then contract with local entities for the actual provision of resettlement services to refugees.

There are two components of refugee resettlement services in the United States. One is reception services; the other is resettlement services. The resettlement funds are restricted in that 85% of these funds must be used for employment-related services. The result has been the creation of a parallel employment assistance program for refugees. The Office of Refugee Resettlement also makes available to the states targeted assistance discretionary grants, under the Refugee Resettlement Program, that are aimed specifically at addressing the needs of localities which are heavily impacted by refugee populations. These funds are awarded on a competitive basis and include monies to provide an incentive for the states to fund self-help, indigenous organizations (often referred to as Mutual Assistance Associations).

Historically, social services to immigrants and refugees were provided through private, nonprofit organizations, usually under the purview of religious entities. Currently, much the same structure exists with the exception that today, the bulk of service delivery in these agencies is provided by paid professional staff instead of volunteers (Ostrander, 1985, p. 435). The government, having assumed the responsibility for provision of services to refugees, has opted for contracting of these services to voluntary agencies. This trend toward government contracting with private agencies to provide social services has resulted in an unclear distinction between public and private sectors (Ibid., p. 436). Nationally, there are approximately 12-13 such agencies serving refugees. At the national level the Office of Refugee Resettlement contracts with these agencies for reception services. For resettlement services, the local branches of these agencies contract with individual states. The three largest resettlement voluntary agencies are the United States Catholic Conference, the Young Men's Christian Association, and the Church World Service.

The Immigration Reform and Control Act (IRCA) of 1986 marked a new era in United States immigration policy. Following over two decades of liberal immigration policy, IRCA signaled the beginning of what might be termed an enforcement period. The IRCA had six major provisions:

1. "A legalization program providing amnesty for undocumented immigrants who meet certain requirements;
2. A program for H-2 temporary foreign workers and seasonal agricultural workers;

3. Employer sanctions penalizing employers who knowingly hire illegal immigrants'' (Espenshade, 1988, p. 4);
4. Anti-discrimination employment provisions;
5. Increased Immigration and Naturalization Service enforcement capabilities; and
6. State Legalization Impact Assistance Grants (SLIAG).

Although all of these provisions are noteworthy, the SLIAG component of the 1986 immigration legislation is of particular relevance. Section 204 of Pub. L. 99-603, the Immigration Reform and Control Act, established SLIAG as a four year mechanism to reimburse "the costs incurred by state and local governments in providing public assistance, public health assistance, and educational services to eligible legalized aliens, as defined in the Act" (Federal Register, 1988, p. 7832). These costs were anticipated as a result of the adjustment of immigration status (from undocumented to documented) by certain groups of aliens residing in the United States. The SLIAG is also under the aegis of the Refugee Resettlement Program. States must request reimbursement by submitting applications to HHS, and "only costs associated with providing services or benefits to eligible legalized aliens, i.e., those granted lawful resident status under sections 245A, 210, and 210A of the Immigration and Nationality Act, may be claimed under SLIAG" (Office of Refugee Resettlement, 1988, p. 3). These requests must be submitted annually, with documentation of incurred expenditures.

The number of individuals applying for adjustment of their legal status to that of temporary resident alien (over three million) is greater than the total number of legal refugees who have entered the country since 1975.[1] As a result, much concern was expressed regarding the potential burden on the states to provide health, education, and social services to this newly legalized population. California, Texas, New York, Florida and Illinois accounted for approximately 85% of the amnesty applications. "The success of registration efforts varied throughout the United States. For example, Texas and California accounted for 70 percent of the 1,533,387 applications filed" (Finch, 1990, p. 250).

For the most part, circumstances which result in the creation of displaced populations are chaotic and unpredictable. Management, by its very definition, is concerned with the ability to control, plan, organize, direct, and predict. The coexistence of these two phenomena within the same organizational system appears to be paradoxical, if not antithetical. The reactive approach required in managing the needs of displaced populations (crisis management) often focuses on their immediate safety and well-being, and frequently fails to acknowledge and support the broader macro management structure. Technology has allowed the human face of the refugee's plight to be transmitted into our homes by mass media. Like the mass media, the social work literature in the area of refugee issues tends to focus on the micro level aspects of service delivery to displaced populations entering the United States.

SOCIAL WORK LITERATURE
ON IMMIGRANTS AND REFUGEES

In reviewing the social work literature, the predominant theme is the refugee as a consumer or recipient of social services. Within this role, there are a number of recurrent issues. First, the barriers and obstacles in service delivery related to language and cultural differences (Mokuau, 1987; Tung, 1985; Weil, 1983). Second, services to refugee youth (unaccompanied minors and international adoptions), and special issues related to elderly refugee populations (Mortland, 1987; Lee, 1987; Metress, 1985). Third, acculturation-assimilation issues experienced by refugees and immigrants (Brodsky, 1988; Bromley, 1987; Tran & Roosevelt, 1987). Fourth, papers highlighting particular aspects of current immigration policy (Finch, 1990). Finally, the literature on refugees focuses primarily on Southeast Asians. Although barriers to social service delivery at the individual and group levels, and general immigration policy issues are discussed; the literature on management issues in the delivery of social services to refugees and immigrants is unavailable.

The objective of this paper is to contribute to the identification of salient issues related to the administration of the social service delivery system for refugees and immigrants. This will be accomplished by focusing on four broad management concerns: funding, service delivery, staffing, and management information needs.

MANAGEMENT ISSUES

Government resettlement services to refugees and immigrants are provided primarily under the purview of Voluntary Service Agencies (VOLAGs). The VOLAGs are "non governmental, nonprofit organizations formed independently of state mandate" (Ostrander, 1985, p. 435). Historically, these voluntary agencies functioned independent of state and federal funding. However, since the 1950s, in the area of refugee resettlement services, voluntary agencies have increasingly used federal government funding for the provision of social services to immigrants and refugees as specialized populations. This practice of utilizing government funds to provide social services has been labeled "nonprofit federalism" (Ibid., p. 436).

Management in the public sector is said to differ from management in the private sector in a number of ways. First, it differs in its output or product. That is, outputs distributed by the public sector are primarily focused on providing services intended to promote general social well-being. Whereas, "the outputs distributed by the private sector are composed of consumption goods and investment goods" (Haveman, 1976, p. 7). Second, in the area of social service delivery, management of human service organizations differs in its treatment and perception of the consumer. In the private for-profit sector, management must be concerned with marketing its product to appeal to the demands of the consumer (consumer driven). The public sector addresses consumers' needs as defined by governmental entities. Third, public sector bureaucracies are distinguished from others in that "they work directly with and on people whose attributes they attempt to shape" (Hazenfield, 1983, p. 1). Finally, public social service agencies are mandated by either federal, state or local government. These entities are then responsible for funding, regulating, structuring, and sanctioning the public social services agencies that they have created.

Funding

Federal funding for resettlement services is allocated on an annual basis. The level of appropriation and allocation to the states is ascertained by refugee population estimates which include: (1) the national population figures on refugees who have been in the United States for a designated period of time (three years or less); and (2) the proportion of the refugee population residing in each state. There are a number of difficulties with such a funding process. First, funding is provided on the basis of the government's perception of the refugee's needs versus the refugee's own felt and perhaps actual needs. Such a model in social service funding can be termed elitist. "Elitism implies that public policy does not reflect demands of 'the people' so much as it does the interests and values of the elite" (Dye, 1978, p. 26). Second, a short-term funding mechanism that hinges on unpredictable and fluctuating populations does not contribute to strategic planning efforts that affect system maintenance and social service delivery. Third, there exists no tracking mechanism for secondary migrants (i.e., individuals who relocate once initial reception and resettlement services have been delivered). This may lead to inflation of the state refugee population estimates, and ultimately, may result in misappropriation of funds. Fourth, innovative program planning and service provision for refugees are limited in that the funding must be applied to meeting needs in the areas of early employment, English language training, and case management services. These services reflect the U.S. Congressional objective that "employable refugees should be placed in jobs as soon as possible after their arrival in the United States" (Federal Register, 1989, p. 19954). Furthermore, the availability of services varies according to the number of refugees eligible to participate in these programs. The entry of a large number of refugees, such as the influx of individuals from Viet Nam, Laos, and Cambodia in the middle 1970s; and the Haitians and Cubans in 1980, is directly correlated with the number of resettlement programs available.

The majority of voluntary agencies in existence today have expanded their service boundaries, and offer a multitude of specialized services that are frequently not available through governmental social service organizations. This specialization, often times with difficult populations, has enhanced their ability to respond to the unique and changing needs of refugee and immigrant populations. Voluntary agencies have gained experience not only in surviving a turbulent refugee service funding environment, but have also developed creative mechanisms for addressing emergent funding issues. One such strategy has been the triangulation of funding sources which has decreased their reliance on federal funding.

As indicated earlier, annual funding; constraints on how the funds are expended; changing, unpredictable refugee numbers; and navigating the federal and state funding allocation mechanisms all create a tempestuous environment. This requires management strategies which are highly tolerant of chaos and ambiguity.

Service Delivery

The access and utilization of public discretionary and entitlement social service programs by noncitizens, legal and illegal, has long been an area of concern. The rights of noncitizens to public benefits are complex and variable, both in the eligibility for, and availability of, services. That is "each program, even those administered at the same level of government, treats alien entitlement differently. This difference in treatment is due primarily to social service law having evolved in a piecemeal fashion from agency to agency" (National Center for Immigrant's Rights, 1986, p. 107). Additionally, citizenship status and classification often entitles individuals to "one benefit and excludes them from others" (Ibid.).

The needs of refugees and immigrants (e.g., eligible legalized aliens) entering and residing in the United States vary, and range from incidental to life threatening. As mentioned earlier, social services for refugee populations are categorized as either reception or resettlement services. Reception services are short-term and immediate, whereas resettlement services are primarily employment-related and are relatively long-term in nature.

The trauma of forced transition is often manifested in adjustment problems experienced both by individuals and by groups. Adjustment problems may not appear during the reception period when the focus by voluntary agencies is on the provision of basic services such as health screening, housing, transportation, and English-as-a-second-language (ESL) training. For instance, "it has been found that . . . after the initial period, emotional and psychological problems begin to appear and the need for mental health counseling becomes apparent" (Tabayas & Pok, 1983, p. 13). Two conflicts are readily apparent. First, eligibility for reception and resettlement services is time-limited, and manifested adjustment problems may be not addressed because their onset occurs after the designated reception period. This situation is exacerbated by the already limited availability of mental health resources for low income populations. The argument that refugee individuals and populations are at risk cannot be overstated. However, their needs are "not always being met, since the services are not always appropriate or even acceptable to this population" (Tung, 1985, p. 5). Second, as mentioned earlier, federal funding requires that refugee social services contribute to rapid "self-sufficiency" (i.e., early employment). Even if adjustment problems were to manifest during the reception period, only 15% of the federal funds would be available for what are considered non-employment related services, such as mental health counseling.

The creation of State Legalization Impact Assistance Grants posed a unique problem for voluntary agencies and other entities involved in social service delivery to refugees and eligible legalized aliens. Admission criteria to the United States as an immigrant includes assurances that the individual will not become a public charge. This is especially salient to the recent eligible legalized alien population since utilization of social services could result in "exclusion" based on the Immigration and Naturalization Service public charge criteria (e.g., not allowed to adjust their status to that of naturalized U.S. citizen). However, with the creation of SLIAG, states can request reimbursement for providing "public assistance, public health assistance, and educational services" to eligible legalized aliens (Federal Register, 1988, p. 7832). This creates an interesting dilemma. On the one hand, SLIAG has increased the likelihood that states will encourage social service utilization among eligible legalized aliens. On the other hand, social service utilization by eligible legalized aliens could jeopardize their immigration status.

Staffing

The exceptional needs which surface in the delivery of social services to refugees and eligible legalized aliens will be the third theme discussed in this article. The ideal, in any situation requiring delivery of social services, is the availability of a well-trained staff. Most managers of refugee reception and resettlement programs would prefer direct service staff who come from similar cultural, racial, ethnic, and linguistic backgrounds. Given the composition of the social work labor force, white, female, young, and middle class (Hardcastle, 1987), there is some question as to whether the needs of refugees and eligible legalized aliens can be effectively understood or addressed. On the one hand, although competency in a foreign language provides access to another culture, it does not guarantee familiarity with that culture. Alternately, the mere familiarity with another language and culture is inadequate, if the worker lacks awareness of the social work knowledge and value base. Management systems must include creative strategies for dealing with these issues.

Language and cultural barriers in social service delivery to refugees have resulted in the utilization of a number of management strategies. Among these are the hiring of professionally trained English-speaking direct service staff, and indigenous bilingual interpreters as support staff; the hiring of paraprofessional bilingual staff; and the reliance on volunteers from the refugee/eligible legalized alien community to serve as interpreters. Each of these solutions is accompanied by a unique set of issues. First, the number of formally trained, certified/licensed social work professionals interested in social service delivery to refugees at the direct service level is very small. Second, voluntary agencies are limited in the financial rewards and long-term employment security they are prepared to offer these individuals.

Second, the introduction of a third person (e.g., the interpreter) in the delivery of social services creates a unique set of problems which must be addressed by management. With the influx of each refugee group into the United States, indigenous staff are recruited and hired by voluntary agencies and other social service providers for what are usually temporary, part-time positions. Management must then resolve the question of human resource utilization. That is, given limited resources, what can be done to develop career ladders for both interpreters and paraprofessionals from refugee and eligible legalized alien communities. Often, many of the refugees hired to assist in or provide social services "have only recently, within a few years, experienced for themselves the traumas of relocation and resettlement" (Wong, 1985, p. 349). Paramount are the development of clear job descriptions, training of social service staff and interpreters in the dynamics of "team" intervention strategies, and monitoring the effectiveness of the team approach.

Third, utilization of volunteers from the eligible legalized aliens and refugee community must be based on sound agency policy and programming which encompasses recruitment, training, monitoring and recognition as essential components. Finally, hiring should not be done in a piecemeal fashion. Long-term strategies and support systems which facilitate further training and certification of "indigenous" social workers should be implemented.

Management Information Needs

In social service delivery to refugees and eligible legalized aliens, management must rely on accurate information for dealing with policy, planning and practice issues. For instance, the importance of a management information system emerged as a major issue with the enactment of State Legalization Impact Assistance Grants (SLIAG). The Immigration Reform and Control Act of 1986 (IRCA) included the provision that "beginning on October 1, 1988, States are required to verify, through Immigration and Nationality Service the legal status of aliens applying for certain public assistance programs (including AFDC and Medicaid)" (Office of Refugee Resettlement, 1988).[2] As mentioned previously, SLIAG is a federal program designed to reimburse states for provision of certain social, health and educational services to newly-legalized aliens. States' requests for reimbursements must have been based on criteria outlined in the SLIAG provisions. One such provision required that states identify specific units of service provided to newly legalized aliens. Until the enactment of IRCA, the majority of state and local social services agencies did not collect citizenship information, and the lack of a mechanism for gathering this and other information on newly legalized aliens has hindered efforts by states in policy and program planning.

CONCLUSION

There are obviously other issues of concern in the management of human service organizations that relate to the effective and efficient delivery of services to refugees and immigrants. These should include "a service delivery model and program orientation that deals with issues related to refugee integration and supportive of cultural pluralism" (Weil, 1983, p. 159). The efficacy of such a model depends on management systems that are aware of and deal creatively with the funding, staffing, service delivery, and the information system needs. "The United States will continue to receive significant numbers of asylum seekers as long as conditions that make people desperate enough to risk the perils of difficult journeys by sea or land continue" (Silk, 1986, p. 44). Therefore, it is imperative that attention be directed to the management of the complex system responsible for the provision of services to these individuals.

NOTES

1. Under the Immigration Reform and Control Act of 1986, amnesty provisions for adjustment to citizenship status entailed three phases:
   Phase I–Registration and adjustment of status to temporary resident.
   Phase II–Participation in English-as-a-second language (ESL) classes and civics training.
   Phase III–Citizenship application and interview.
2. This could be waived if it was found not to be cost-effective or if a State had an alternative system that is as effective and timely as that mandated by the Immigration Reform and Control Act.

REFERENCES

Adler, P.M. (1985). Ethnic placement of refugee/entrant unaccompanied minors. *Child Welfare, 64*(5), 491-499.

Brodsky, B. (1988). Mental health attitudes and practices of Soviet Jewish immigrants. *Health and Social Work, 13*(2), 130-136.

Bromley, M.A. (1987). New beginnings for Cambodian refugees–or further disruptions. *Social Work, 32*(3), 236-239.

Dye, T.R. (1978). *Understanding public policy* (3rd Edition). New Jersey: Prentice-Hall, Inc.

Espenshade, T. J.; et al., (1988). *Immigration policy in the United States: Future prospects for the Immigration Reform and Control Act of 1986.* Washington D.C.; The Urban Institute.

Federal Register (1990, June 27). State Legalization Impact Assistance Grants. *Rules and Regulations, 55*(124), 26206-26207.

Federal Register (1989, May 23). Refugees resettlement program: Allocations to states of FY 1989 funds for refugee social services. *Notices, 54*(88), 19954-19958.

Federal Register (1988, March 10). State Legalization Impact Assistance Grants; Final rule. *Rules and Regulations, 53*(47), 7832-7833.

Finch, W. A. (1990). The immigration reform and control act of 1986: A preliminary assessment. *Social Service Review, 64*(2), 243-260.

Hardcastle, D. A. (1987). *The social work labor force.* Texas: School of Social Work, University of Texas at Austin.

Haveman, R. H. (1976). *The economics of the public sector* (2nd Edition). New York: John Wiley & Sons, Inc.

Hazenfeld, Y (1983). *Human service organizations.* New Jersey: Prentice-Hall, Inc.

Le-Doux, C.C. (1987). *United States immigration policy and social service provision for immigrants.* Unpublished manuscript, School of Social Work, University of Texas at Austin.

Lee, J. (1987). Asian American elderly: A neglected minority group. *Ethnicity and Gerontological Social Work,* 103-116.

Metress, S. P. (1985). The history of Irish-American care of the aged. *Social Service Review, 59*(1), 18-31.

Mokuau, N. (1987). Social workers' perceptions of counseling effectiveness for Asian American clients. *Social Work, 32*(4), 331-335.

Mortland, C.A. & Egan, M.G. (1987). Vietnamese youth in American foster care. *Social Work, 32*(3), 240-245.

National Center for Immigrant's Rights (1986). *Immigration and naturalization law* (2nd Edition). Los Angeles, CA: Author.

Office of Refugee Resettlement (1988). *The State Legalization Impact Assistance Grants: Program Implementation Workshop.* Sponsored by the U.S. Department of Health and Human Services, Austin, TX, March 22-23.

Ostrander, S.A. (1985). Voluntary social service agencies in the United States. *Social Service Review, 59*(3), 435-454.

Silk, J. (1986). *Despite a Generous spirit: Denying asylum in the United States.* Washington, D C: American Council for Nationalities Service (ISSN 00882-9276).

Tayabas, T. & Pok, T. (1983). The Southeast Asian refugee's arrival in America: An overview. In Special Service for Groups, *Bridging cultures: Social work with Southeast Asian refugees* (pp. 3-14). Los Angeles, CA: Asian American Community Mental Health Training Center (Author).

Tran, T. V., Roosevelt, W., Jr., & Mindel, C. H. (1987). Alienation among Vietnamese refugees in the United States: A causal approach. *Journal of Social Service Research, 11*(1), 59-75.

Tran, T. V. & Wright, R., Jr., (1986). Social support and subjective well-being among Vietnamese refugees. *Social Service Review, 60*(3), 449-459.
Tung, T. M. (1985). Psychiatric care for Southeast Asians: How different is different? In. T.C. Owan (Ed.), *Southeast Asian mental health: Treatment, prevention, services, training, and research* (pp. 5-40). DC: U.S. Department of Health and Human Services (NIMH).
Weil, M. (1983). Southeast Asians and service delivery–Issues in service provision and institutional racism. In Special Service for Groups, *Bridging cultures: Social work with Southeast Asian refugees* (pp. 136-163). Los Angeles, CA: Asian American Community Mental Health Training Center (Author).
Wong, H. Z. (1985). Training for mental health service providers to Southeast Asian refugees: Models, strategies, and curricula. In. T.C. Owan (Ed.), *Southeast Asian mental health: Treatment, prevention, services, training, and research* (pp. 354-390). Washington, DC: U.S. Department of Health and Human Services (NIMH).

Integration and Xenophobia:
An Inherent Conflict
in International Migration

Nazneen S. Mayadas
Doreen Elliott

SUMMARY. This paper addresses issues in the settlement of immigrant and refugee groups and discusses the concept of xenophobia (fear of foreigners) as a key factor in inhibiting integration of the newcomers with the dominant host society. A paradigm is proposed for the analysis and assessment of the type and level of integration achieved by various incoming groups. The model looks at immigrants on two dimensions of integration: economic and cultural, and provides four cells for classification: Assimilation, Accommodation, Adaptation and Alienation. The paper argues that economic variables are a primary influence in facilitating integration and reducing xenophobia.

It is one of the tragedies of our age that people who have left their own countries to escape from persecution and prejudice should suffer from exactly the same evils in the countries to which they have fled.

–Raymond Hall. Refugees *81*, 1990:31

This paper examines the relocation problems of immigrants and refugees settling in industrialized countries and suggests a framework for analyzing factors affecting their integration.

Nazneen S. Mayadas, DSW, is Professor, and Doreen Elliott, PhD, is Associate Professor at The University of Texas at Arlington, Graduate School of Social Work, Arlington, TX 76019.

The influx of immigrants and refugees into the west presents a significant social problem. For example, South East Asian Refugees arriving in the U.S.A. numbered approximately 846,000 from 1975-87 (As reported by the Office of Refugee Resettlement in 1988). A 1987 report informs that of the 50,000 Ethiopians in the U.S.A., 15,000 qualify as refugees (Refugees, 1987, 44:17-18). Over the last thirty years, more than 800,000 Cuban refugees have settled in Florida (Refugees, 1990: 79,28). To date, 3.9 million illegal aliens have been estimated in the U.S.A. Of these 550,000-600,000 are Salvadorans; 150,000-200,000 are Nicaraguans (Refugees 1987: 45, 9-10), with other smaller groups representing Guatemalans and Mexicans from the Latin world. Haitians and Cubans from the Caribbean, and from Asia, Taiwan, Hong Kong, Korea, the Philippines, China, as well as the Middle East, Africa, India, Pakistan, and Europe (Refugees 1987: 42, 12). Notwithstanding language, these newcomers differ from nationals in cultural mores, values, and habits as well as being conspicuous, primarily due to differences in physical appearance. Both the continued influx and these differences contribute to xenophobic reactions amongst nationals, who are both emotionally and intellectually unable to grasp their governments' "open-door" policies to offer asylum and resettlement opportunities to people who look, and are, different, and thus are perceived as posing a threat to the nation's solidarity. The newcomers experience this xenophobic reaction as institutionalized discrimination (Beeghley, 1989:77).

XENOPHOBIA

Xenophobia is defined as a basic fear and contempt of foreigners; it is the self-centered egocentricity of human kind against people who are different (Refugees, 12:1984;), and as such fall into the category of outsiders.

Xenophobia has both social-structural and interpersonal components and operates at a number of levels:

- *National Policies* impact world immigration patterns. The majority of refugees from developing nations are relocated within other developing countries (Zolberg et al., 1989). For example, 6,773,365 refugees are in Asia and 4,587,272 in

Africa as opposed to 1,380,200 in North America and 745,225 in Europe (Refugees, 1989, 71:22). Popular opinion in many industrialized nations is ignorant of this fact, and contains myths believing that the resettlement countries are bearing the major burden of immigration patterns worldwide. National governments operate gatekeeping policies, fixing national quotas which sometimes suffer from "compassion fatigue" (Refugees, 12:1984). For example, with the total world population of refugees reaching the 15 million mark, the USA had set a ceiling of 125,000 for resettlement as of October 1989. (Refugees 1989, 71:28).

- *Nationalism* is fostered in many countries, e.g., in the U.S.A. where school children recite the pledge and controversy over flag-burning raises high feeling. The recent revival of nationalism in Europe has been clearly evident. Nationalism may serve to forge a strong identity, but its unacceptable face manifests itself in popular belief systems and ideologies where the outsider is always stigmatized and often, especially in times of economic recession, scapegoated.

- *Institutionalized discrimination* in the social structure occurs when it becomes clear that a society discriminates in the access which different racial groups have to societal resources such as income, employment, education, health and social services (DiNitto and Dye, 1983; Ginsburg, 1989). Indigenous minority as well as immigrant groups suffer from this form of discrimination.

- *Lack of accommodation* on the part of resettlement countries exhibits itself as a form of passive aggression to the outsiders. For example, refugee resettlement programs in many western industrialized countries offer only short term support, and are characteristically residual in nature (Mayadas and Elliott, 1990). The immigrant is thrown on the existing structures which either fail to accommodate or are discriminatory.

- *Interpersonal prejudice*: in this component of xenophobia, fear of the foreigner, cultural and religious differences, social boundaries, economic insecurity and popular ideologies all contribute to prejudice which may be expressed on a personal basis by rejection of outsiders, and in some cases, violence and aggression towards them.

50 Social Work with Immigrants and Refugees

Whilst indigenous minority groups are victimized by *institution-alized discrimination, lack of accommodation* and *interpersonal prejudice,* they participate in the country's spirit of *nationalism* and support of *national policies* which may adversely affect immigrants and refugees. Hence the xenophobic reactions extended to foreigners has the additional element of resentment towards strangers. Thus discrimination exists on the basis of race, age, gender, education, etc. but does not necessarily entail xenophobia. Put another way, xenophobia subsumes discrimination, whilst discrimination can exist independently of xenophobia.

An example of xenophobia is the policy of "humane deterrence" which is based on the position that detention of refugees acts as a control mechanism for the future inflow of asylees (Eggs, 1984). The assumption made here is that once refugees recognize that they will be maintained under prison like conditions in the asylum country for indefinite periods, they will be unlikely to flee their own country and seek asylum. As a function of this stance, closed asylum camps have been set up in some Asian countries, e.g., in Hong Kong the closed camp policy was activated in July 1982, when asylum seekers from Vietnam were placed under the authority of the penitentiary department, in abandoned prison buildings on remote islands, accessible only by patrol boats (Eggs, 1984). Refugees who find themselves in these circumstances realize that they have defied mortal danger to escape persecution, only to endure indefinite confinement.

Another example of xenophobic behavior is the attitude of certain sea captains, when seafaring vessels ignore cries for help from the "boat people" on the high seas, since international law requires that the country under whose flag the ship is sailing is to provide asylum to the rescued. The captain may base his judgement on his assessment of his country's attitude towards asylees, and on his own prejudices. Whatever his rationale may be, the result is the destruction of humankind.

A third example from the international scene is that of Malaysia, where Vietnamese Boat People are "pushed off" to other neighboring countries. A recent report suggests that 5,561 such asylum seekers were turned away, despite the dire condition of their boats and their poor physical state (Refugees, 76:1990).

Other examples of xenophobia include the recent restrictions introduced in the immigration policies of the U.S.A. (Refugees, 41:1987) where legislation was amended to support non-deportation of asylum seekers, but evidence of persecution in the home country was made mandatory, leaving many people with an indeterminate status (Goodwin-Gill, 1987) and Australia where new rules have been introduced to narrow the criteria for giving residence on humanitarian grounds (Refugees, 74:1990). The resurgence of nationalism in Europe (Refugees, 74:1990) and the continuance of attacks on the sea of Vietnamese Boat People in South East Asia (Refugees, 76:1990) also have a xenophobic component.

The above situations are but a few examples of the xenophobic reactions which refugees may encounter during their initial attempt to seek refuge. This reaction takes on a more subtle form during the interim stage of asylum camps, where refugees await selection by resettlement countries. Periods of wait are interminably long, because western countries are reluctant to admit refugees, as they are suffering from "compassion fatigue" (Refugees, 12:1984). Intake quotas are way down as compared to the 1975-79 period. As one camp manager stated (Eggs, 1984), "only about 10-20% of a boatload will ever be resettled–the others have no chance of leaving the prison-like camp conditions." Refugees who do make it to the country of resettlement face a whole new set of xenophobic reactions which for many may frequently be a life long ordeal.

Immigrating groups comprise not only persons who have been victimized by political or religious persecution, but also include economic migrants in search of lifestyles consistent with their own expectational goals. Regardless of the causal factors, this influx of newcomers into a country is perceived by nationals as putting a strain on cultural homogeneity, threatening to established societal norms. This is more so, if existing patterns are disrupted and new norms emerge to contradict traditional values. The repercussions of this change are felt both by the national and by the immigrant refugee, and frequently results are not in the best interest of either party (Stern, 1981). Moreover, if the receiving country itself is in the throes of an economic recession, the reception of strangers who look, act and speak differently is often viewed by nationals as a violation of their rights. They seem to be at a loss to understand why the age-old adage "charity begins at home" is, in their view, no longer a priority of their government. This instinct of self-preservation (often manifested as nationalism) compounded by the lack of a global perspective amongst the populace, often results in conditions detrimental to the newcomers. For the immigrant, xenophobic reactions can result in loneliness, communication problems, accommodation scarcity, lack of employment or work much below the immigrants' skill level, and a general sense of constantly living on the periphery of society. Mass xenophobia, therefore, occurs when government policies towards refugees and migrants and the attitude of the general public towards them, do not match. While the selection of refugees for resettlement denotes political and legal recognition by the government, it does not serve as a passport to social acceptance by the nationals (Refugees, 50:1988). Nor does it serve as a passport to economic success. The acceptance problems of the new immigrant are compounded by inadequate resettlement policies, and programs which are piecemeal and operate only for a brief period after arrival. One resolution of this situation is to extend national resettlement schemes to include integration programs for refugees until such time as they reach a minimum level of economic stability–a prerequisite to social acceptance, and an antidote for xenophobia. A national concerted effort on the part of the country concerned would be more effective than the present piecemeal action by voluntary organizations or refugees being left to their own devices (Crisp, 1988).

Economic status is a key factor in refugee resettlement. One recent illustration is the Canadian and British Governments' policy of accepting only those immigrants from Hong Kong whose resources are available for self support and investment. The importance placed here on economic status is ironic when the definition of the term refugee is considered. This was politically defined by western nations after World War II to resettle selected groups of Europeans. It has since then been maintained as a selective term, and has always excluded economic migrants (Mayadas and Elliott, 1990). In the U.S.A., South East Asians, Ethiopians, and asylees from Communist countries are recognized as refugees, but Salvadoreans are not (Refugees 1987: *45*, 9-10), based on the view the U.S.A. government takes of the respective country's political regime (Refugees, 1987: *41*, 8-10).

In summary, xenophobic reactions stem from a composite base which may be attributed to social, political, religious, cultural and psychological factors. Mayadas and Lasan (1984) advocate a dual faceted approach directed both at the individual and social change. This paper extends it further and suggests that a multifaceted approach is needed to counter this malaise.

FRAMEWORK FOR ANALYSIS

This paper argues the importance of socio-economic structural issues and institutional discrimination, and suggests that key issues in resettlement and integration are the dimension of economic advantage/disadvantage and cultural identity. Two classes of variables are isolated as predictors of xenophobia, i.e., socio-economic status (which includes class, education, age and gender) and cultural identity (which includes language, religion, rituals, values, dress, food, art, music political affiliation). While all these discriminatory factors may be experienced by indigenous minority groups, the immigrant experiences additional xenophobic reactions which cover a broader range of discriminatory practices.

The following paradigm is offered as a framework for understanding levels and degrees of immigrant integration into the host society.

Integration is viewed on a two dimensional axis (Figure I). The horizontal axis represents a continuum from high economic integration to low economic integration, while the vertical axis represents high and low cultural integration. The resulting four cells represent positions which have been called Assimilation, Accommodation, Adaptation and Alienation.

Cell A: Assimilation

This position is characterized by high economic as well as high cultural integration, and may be achieved by first generation immigrants from similar cultures or by second generations onwards from cultures whose language, values and religion may be very different from the dominant host culture. In some cases it may be a slow evolutionary process and span many generations, e.g., as in

FIGURE I: INTEGRATION ASSESSMENT PARADIGM

Cultural Integration
+
HI

CELL A   ASSIMILATION: Very low xenophobia
                       Very low discrimination

High economic & high cultural integration
into dominant majority culture.
Characterized by:
—above average income
—1st generation immigrants from Western
  industrialized countries
—2nd generation immigration from other
  countries

ADAPTATION: Low xenophobia   CELL C
            High discrimination

High cultural and low economic integration.
Characterized by:
—institutionalized
  discrimination
—poor skills, poor education
—culturally adopted values, norms and
  aspiration of dominant culture.
—mostly indigenous minority groups

Economic
+ HI——LO –
Integration   Integration

CELL B   ACCOMODATION: Low xenophobia
                        Low discrimination

Economically integrated minority
sub-cultures, characterized by:
—Public integration, personal ethnic
  identity
—cultural pluralism
—permeable boundaries
—development
—acceptance of change
—first generation professionals

ALIENATION: Very high xenophobia   CELL D
            Very high discrimination

Immigrant groups remain outsiders economically
and culturally. Barriers to change:
—language, religion
—impermeable boundaries
—resistance to change
—xenophobia, institutionalized
  discrimination
—rural tribal groups
—ghetto dwellers, elderly, women

LO
–
Cultural
Integration

Summary of chart

CELL A	High Economic Integration ⟩	Very low xenophobia
	High Cultural Integration ⟩	Very low discrimination
CELL B	High Economic Integration ⟩	Low xenophobia
	Low Cultural Integration ⟩	Low discrimination
CELL C	Low Economic Integration ⟩	Low xenophobia
	High Cultural Integration ⟩	High discrimination
CELL D	Low Economic Integration ⟩	Very high xenophobia
	Low Cultural Integration ⟩	Very high discrimination

Britain and in the U.S.A. where over hundreds of years different nationalities have combined to form a relatively homogenous group, which in turn may reject more recent immigrants. However, Beeghley (1989) suggests that ethnic inequality decreases as educational attainment, occupational prestige and subsequent income level increase, indicating social acceptability and integration into the majority group. Parks (1950) proposed that the natural evolution of ethnic/race relations was towards assimilation. However, Parks probably underestimated the importance of the economic dimension, for he was not to know that nearly forty years later, 31.8% of African-American families and 27.7% of Hispanic families in America would be in poverty, compared with only 9.1% of white families (U.S. Bureau of Census, 1989). That some immigrants do achieve assimilation is attested by those who become public figures, and those in the professions and large corporations, who clearly are integrated in both cultural and economic aspects of American life. The experience of immigrants in this cell would suggest that economic status and social class is a more powerful predictor of discrimination than race. Groups represented in this cell would be:

- First generation immigrants from the western industrialized world.
- High economic status second generation immigrants from the developing countries.
- Professionals and high economic status persons from indigenous ethnic minority groups.
- Individual defectors from communist countries, e.g., tennis players, musicians, gymnasts, etc.

Cell B: Accommodation

Groups in this cell are high on the economic ladder but choose to maintain their cultural uniqueness. They are economically integrated, and project a public image of accommodating to the dominant culture, in that they reside in upper middle class neighborhoods, and are high achievers in professions and other work fields. However, in their personal lives, they prefer an ethnic social milieu. An example is the Asian Indian minority in the U.S.A. Accommodation is conceptualized as a process of integration, characterized by structural and cultural pluralism (Steinberg, 1989), permeable boundaries across which awareness of the majority and minority cultures may be acquired, and an open acceptance of differences by varying systemic levels, i.e., governmental, institutional, community and individual. Persons in this category, though racially different bear socio-economic similarity to the dominant culture. These persons may not directly experience xenophobic and discriminatory reactions, but remain potential victims, depending on the level of tolerance for pluralism in the majority culture. This group consists of first generation professionals from developing countries, such as Asians and Latin Americans, who have immigrated to the U.S.A. as individuals through legal channels. They select to live in integrated upper middle class neighborhoods but tenaciously maintain their cultural preference.

Cell C: Adaptation

Persons in this cell are culturally adapted to the majority culture, but the institutional structures of the system are not geared to adapt to their economic condition. They lack opportunity for education, skills training and gainful employment. Having strong identification with the majority culture, they share the same values, norms and aspirations of the dominant group, but are denied the means to achieve these through lack of social and economic opportunities. Persons who fall into this cell would be members of indigenous groups, such as Puerto Ricans, African Americans or ethnic immigrants who have been in the country over generations, but have a history of socio-economic oppression. This group suffers high discrimination but does not provoke a significant xenophobic reaction.

Cell D: Alienation

Groups in this cell consist of individuals who due to various endogenous and exogenous factors are left to their own devices. These groups perforce are separated from mainstream society and lack means of integration. They are characterized by cultural segregation and impermeable boundaries which preclude any significant interactional exchange outside their own milieu. The insular nature of their existence makes them resistant to change and through xenophobic reaction they become victims of prejudice. They are caught in a vicious circle caused by stereotyped patterns of reactions and institutionalized racism towards them which in turn produces more defensive and insular behaviors, thus reinforcing the separatist position. Persons in this group are discriminated against for lack of language and skills, and on the basis of age and gender. Groups such as the rural tribal people from Laos, Hmongs and Laotians (Yu & Mayadas, 1990); Ghetto dwellers (Segal, 1991) and elderly women attached to extended families with no exposure to integration skills, fall into this category.

FRAMEWORK FOR INTERVENTION

In order to enable immigrants who are locked into social situations corresponding to cells C and D in Figure I, responses are required of the dominant culture which will address the economic and social structural issues embodied in the concept of xenophobia and which work to the disadvantage of these groups. Four levels of responses may be identified: policy, institutional, community and individual.

Policy

The policies of immigration are among the most politically sensitive issues with which governments have to deal. Immigrants are generally over-represented among the poorest and most disadvantaged groups in society. Ethnic minority groups are substantially over-represented in the number of unemployed; children in public care; men in prison; juveniles appearing before the courts, and in the economically poorest groups in society (Karger & Stoesz, 1990). Policies of positive discrimination have been inhibited by positions on all points of the political spectrum. Socialists argue that all disadvantaged groups need extra help and that policies involving redistribution of resources within society (e.g., by higher taxation) will best serve the interests of the disadvantaged, irrespective of racial origin. Liberals argue that positive discrimination leads to separate services and identify separation with segregation and as such see it as inimical to the rights of the individual. Conservative policy focuses on severe restriction on public spending. All political groups have therefore tended to emphasize positions which inhibit the development of specialist services for minorities. Conservative policies in both Britain and the U.S.A., which have resulted in severe cutbacks in welfare expenditure have a proportionately greater effect on immigrant groups because of their large numbers in the poorer classes.

Institutions

The large scale failure of institutions such as welfare, social, health and education services to respond to immigrant groups is strikingly evident, since the latter are often poor and unskilled, and suffer ill health, yet they make proportionately fewer demands on these services than those made by the general population. For example, studies of referrals to social service departments in Britain (e.g., Jackson, 1981; Horn, 1982) show that the proportion of Asian families referred to, or referring themselves to social service departments and special services such as day nurseries is far below that in the general population.

Discrimination in job interviews, applications for home mortgages and racial prejudice by the police are further examples of institutional racism (Campling, 1986a). Another example common to both the U.S.A. and the U.K. is the provision of meals on wheels service and the emphasis on providing food according to the eating traditions of the dominant culture. Institutional change is notoriously slow, and will occur only through influence from policy on the one hand and local pressure on the other. Concerted efforts are therefore needed to identify problematic institutional responses and to change these appropriately.

One of the most influential institutions in any society in changing attitudes is the media. Representation of minority cultures in the media still remains token. Exposure, bringing about familiarity with another culture is one of the best ways of reducing fear and suspicion, and therefore xenophobia. Concerted efforts by the media in this regard have yet to be made.

Negative bias in the media can be seen in various ways: reporting of crime, for instance, needs careful monitoring, because often the ethnic origin of suspects is mentioned only when they come from immigrant groups. This has the effect of reinforcing stereotyped images of immigrants and feeding xenophobic reaction. Just as in the case of political figures, the media has the power to either make or break the image of the immigrants, but as yet this challenge has been ignored.

Community

Many of the policy and institutional issues discussed above are reflected in interaction in local communities. Education can be a major force for changing attitudes of younger majority members, and through adult education programs, for influencing attitudes in the older generation. Interventions at the community level could be designed to (1) relocate immigrants in small numbers in majority neighborhoods, where opportunity exists for face to face interaction; (2) prepare both the neighborhood and the immigrants for mutual acceptance; (3) avoid ghettos, since these reinforce stereotypic myths, and (4) use local institutions such as churches, schools, community centers to involve immigrants and nationals to exchange cultural view points, foods and life styles as an expansion of learning.

Organizations set up to negotiate the boundaries between the new and old cultures are particularly important. In Britain the setting up of Community Relations Councils at a local level has had mixed success. Barker (1981) in a study of these organizations, has identified three models: the *Shelter* assists immigrants with their problems as interpreter, information provider and with advice on rights: the *Bridge* fulfills a coordinating function, providing a meeting place for organizations from different ethnic groups and may act as a stimulator in encouraging communication between them; the *Platform* acts as a campaigning organization, sees its role in consciousness raising, drawing attention to discriminatory practices and may be seen as militant. The role of these councils varies widely in practice, the Bridge may be mainly social, recreational and cultural and the Platform political in style. Few councils have successfully combined all three models.

A key issue in community organizations is that they should act as a stimulator to institutions rather than replace their role in relation to immigrant groups. For example, community organizations in setting up educational activities, must be reminded that their program is not an alternative to the school's assumption of responsibility for curriculum change and for meeting community needs. Community relations alone cannot however change structures for example, minority community leaders should not be blamed for failing to control their youth when it is unemployment, poverty, policing methods and racial discrimination which are the root of the dissatisfaction. Community relations can support, but not replace institutional and policy change.

Individual

The upheavals, traumas and crises experienced by refugees even before arriving in their country of resettlement have been documented in the foregoing discussion. It has been argued that xenophobic reaction on arrival and after settlement creates isolation and numerous other social and psychological problems for the refugees.

Thus working with individuals and families to enable them to deal with their experiences so as to maximize their potential for resettlement, to help them to key into social resources and community networks, and to facilitate education of the other culture in both host and immigrant groups are key tasks for social workers.

Since social work is a change-oriented profession it may be argued that it is well placed to improve the lives of refugees in that its areas of expertise cover the range of systems at social-structural, policy and individual levels which can best help the individual. Other professions may be limited by professional boundaries to operating at one level only, such as education or therapy. The need is clear: social work needs to take on the challenge in a more systematized way. To intervene at all four systemic levels to promote cultural pluralism and economic integration.

REFERENCES

Barker, A. (1981). Strategy and style in local community relations. In J. Cheetham, et al. (Eds.), *Social and community work in a multi-racial society.* London: Harper and Row.
Beeghley, L. (1989). *The structure of social stratification in the United States.* Boston: Allyn and Bacon.
Campling, J. (1986a). Social Administration Digest, *58*, 8.5-8.8, *Journal of Social Policy, 15*(2), 249; Social Administration Digest, *60*, 8.3, *Journal Social Policy, 15*(4), 519.
Campling, J. (1986b). Social Administration Digest, *59*, 8.7, *Journal of Social Policy, 15*(3), 376.
Crisp, J. (1988). New country, new culture, *Refugees.* United Nations High Commissioner for Refugees, 58, 30-32.
DiNitto, D., & Dye, T. R. (1989). *Social welfare: Politics and public policy.* Englewood Cliffs, NJ: Prentice Hall, Inc.
Eggs, M. (1984). Closed camps: a preliminary assessment, *Refugees, 10,* 16.
Ginsburg, N. (1989). Institutional racism and local authority housing. *Critical Social Policy, 24*(8.3), 4-19.
Goodwin-Gill, G. S. (1987). Supreme court rules on asylum. *Refugees, 41,* 8-10. Geneva: United Nations High Commissioner for Refugees.
Hall, R. (1990). Xenophobia: the barometer of intolerance. *Refugees 81:* 29-31. Geneva: United Nations High Commissioner for Refugees.
Horn, B. E. (1982). A survey of referrals from asian families to four social services area offices. In J. Cheetham, (Eds.), *Social work and ethnicity.* London: Allen and Unwin.
Hraba, J. (1979). *American ethnicity.* Itasca, IL: F. E. Peacock.
Jackson, A. (1981). Just how relevant and accessible are social services departments? In J. Cheetham (Ed), *Social work with immigrants.* London & Boston: Routledge and Kegan Paul.
Karger, H. J. & Stoesz, D. (1990). American Social Welfare Policy: A structural approach. New York and London: Longman.
Mayadas, N. S. & Elliott, D. (1990). Refugees: An introductory case-study in international social welfare. In D. Elliott, N. S. Mayadas, & T. D. Watts (Eds.), *The World of Social Welfare: Social Welfare and Services in an International Context* (Chapter 18). Springfield, IL: Charles C Thomas, Publisher.
Mayadas, N. S. & Lasan, D. B. (1984). Integrating refugees into alien cultures. In C. Guzzetta, et al. (Eds.), *Educational for social work practice: Selected international models.* NY: CSWE, II ASSW.
Parks, R. (1950). *Race & culture.* Glencoe, IL: Free Press.
Refugees 12. (1984). Has "compassion fatigue" overtaken the shipping community? *Refugees, 12,* 15-16. Geneva: United Nations High Commissioner for Refugees.
Refugees 41. (1987). Interaction. *Refugees, 41,* 40-41. Geneva: United Nations High Commissioner for Refugees.

Refugees 41. (1987). Supreme Court rules on asylum. *Refugees, 41,* 8-10. Geneva: United Nations High Commissioner for Refugees.
Refugees 42. (1987). Illegals come out of the shadows. *Refugees, 42,* 12-14. Geneva: United Nations High Commissioner for Refugees.
Refugees 44. (1987). Ethiopians in California: aspirations and reality. *Refugees, 41,* 17-18. Geneva: United Nations High Commissioner for Refugees.
Refugees 45. (1987). Boomerang of fortune. *Refugees, 45,* 9-10. Geneva: United Nations High Commissioner for Refugees.
Refugees 50. (1988). A charter for refugees. *Refugees, 50,* 39-40. Geneva: United Nations High Commissioner for Refugees.
Refugees 58. (1988). Yes to a colourful community! *Refugees, 58,* 17-33. Geneva: United Nations High Commissioner for Refugees.
Refugees 71. (1989). Refugee population by continent. *Refugees, 71,* 22. Geneva: United Nations High Commissioner for Refugees.
Refugees 71. (1989). Diverse developments. *Refugees, 71,* 28-29. Geneva: United Nations High Commissioner for Refugees.
Refugees 74. (1990). Interview: Bernard Kouchner. *Refugees, 74,* 14, 40-42. Geneva: United Nations High Commissioner for Refugees.
Refugees 76. (1990). Boat people: A continuing drama. *Refugees, 76,* 11-14. Geneva: United Nations High Commissioner for Refugees.
Refugees 79. (1990). Little Havana. *Refugees, 79,* 28-29. Geneva: United Nations High Commissioner for Refugees.
Report to Congress. (1988, January 31). *Refugee resettlement program.* U.S. Department of Health and Human Service, Office of Refugee Resettlement.
Segal, U. A. (1991). Cultural variables in Asian Indian Families, *Families in Society: The Journal of Contemporary Human Services,* 72,(4), 233-242.
Steinberg, S. (1989). *The ethnic myth: Race, ethnicity and class in America.* Boston: Bacon Press.
Stern, L. M. (1981). Response to vietnamese refugees: Surveys of public opinion, *Social Work, 26*(4), 306-312.
U.S. Bureau of the Census. (1989). Current population reports. Series P-60, No. 163. *Poverty in the United States.* Washington, D.C.: 1987 U.S. Government Printing Office.
Yu, Muriel, & Mayadas, Nazneen S. The micro-systems impact upon the Southeast Asian Refugees and needed Social Work Interventions. Paper presented at the Annual National Association of Social Workers Meeting in Boston, Mass. November 16, 1990.
Zolberg, A. R., Suhrke, A., & Aguayo, S. (1989). *Escape from violence: Conflict and the refugee crisis in the developing world.* New York and Oxford: Oxford University Press.

A Stage of Migration Framework
As Applied to Recent Soviet Emigres

Diane Drachman
Anna Halberstadt

SUMMARY. To facilitate understanding and assistance to immigrant populations, a framework on stages in the migration process is described and applied to recent Soviet emigres in the United States. Practice examples illustrating issues associated with each of the stages in the migration process are presented. Recent changes in Soviet emigration and United States admission policy responses are discussed in light of their implications for individual and family adaptation and service delivery.

This paper presents a conceptual framework on stages in the migration process to facilitate understanding and assistance to immigrant and refugee clients.[1] The framework which is applicable to all immigrant groups (Dewind, 1990; Drachman and Ryan, 1990; Gil, 1990; Mandel, 1990; O and Porr, 1990) will be applied to Soviet emigres in the United States. Practice examples illustrating issues associated with each of the stages in the migration process will be presented. Recent changes in Soviet emigration and United States admission policy responses will be discussed in light of their implications for individual and family adaptation and service delivery. The migration circumstances of Soviet emigres who entered the United States prior to 1986 will be compared to those of recent arrivals.

Diane Drachman, DSW, is Associate Professor at the University of Connecticut School of Social Work. Anna Halberstadt, MSW, is Casework Supervisor of Refugee Assistance Services at the Jewish Board of Family Services, New York.

Diane Drachman's mailing address is University of Connecticut, School of Social Work, 1798 Asylum Avenue, West Hartford, CT 06117.

In recent years there has been a major wave of migration to the United States. According to the United States Census, the foreign born population increased by 46% between the years 1970-1980 (U.S. Census 1970; U.S. Census 1980). The continued rise in immigrant populations has been highlighted in labor force projections for the twenty-first century. One report states that immigrants will represent the largest share of the increase in the population and in the workforce since World War I (Johnston and Packer, 1987).

Soviet emigres, many of whom are Jewish are included in the rising immigrant population. According to the Soviet Jewry Research Bureau, 11,191 Soviet Jews left the Soviet Union in November, 1989–the highest monthly figure since the Bureau began tabulating emigration statistics. (Wall Street Journal, Dec. 13, 1989 p. 10). A large proportion of the individuals have come to the United States (Pear, 1989a). It is expected that 50,000 will arrive in the United States in 1990 (Saperia and Stolow 1989).

Service providers and organizations in contact with Soviet emigres and other newly arriving groups have reported on their needs and the paucity of professionally trained personnel capable of understanding their different cultures, their different migration experiences and the unique issues they face in the process of adjustment to living in the United States. Although understanding and providing service to the culturally diverse new populations is a challenge–the challenge is historically familiar as the social work profession has traditionally applied generic practice knowledge and skills accompanied by the necessary specific information to respond to new groups. "Attention to today's immigrant population requires exactly what has always been necessary–a framework for practice that allows one to learn about the particular needs and circumstances of the new population being served and the methodology and skills to be helpful" (Meyer, 1984, p. 99).

The stage of migration framework outlined in this discussion is responsive to this practice task. It creates a vehicle for workers to obtain knowledge of the needs, experiences, and circumstances of the new and different immigrant groups. It facilitates understanding of changing circumstances in migration such as changes in recent Soviet emigration as well as shifting U.S. admission policies. It is applicable to the individual in the particular situation of migration.

It has utility for direct practice and program planning. Since it is based on the notion that migration is a recurring phenomenon rather than a temporary unique historical event it can be applied to future newcomers (Stein, 1986). It enables practitioners and organizations to take into account similarities and differences in experiences, circumstances and helping approaches for both the past and present immigrant groups. Thus, lessons learned from the past could inform present helping approaches (Drachman, 1990; Drachman and Ryan, 1990).

The framework builds on the work of numerous writers in the field and study of migration who have observed and formulated stages in the migration process (Cox, 1985; Keller, 1975). The framework used in this discussion highlights three phases–pre-migration or departure, transit, and resettlement (Drachman, 1990; Drachman and Ryan, 1990). It is based on the following assumptions. "All immigrants have an experiential past; some experience abrupt departure while others experience a decision-making process and a period of preparation for a move; a physical move is always involved and finally resettlement and some type of adjustment to a new environment occurs" (Cox, 1985, p. 75). Although the framework is emphasized, it is assumed that variables of age, family composition, socioeconomic level, education, culture, occupation, rural or urban background, belief system and social support will interact with the migration process and color the individual or group experience in each of the migration stages (Drachman, 1990; Drachman and Ryan, 1990). Table 1 illustrates the critical variables associated with each phase in the migration process.

PRE-MIGRATION AND DEPARTURE EXPERIENCES

The social political and economic factors surrounding the pre-migration/departure stage are significant. This phase may involve abrupt exile and flight or a situation in which individuals choose to depart but wait for years for permission to exit. Separation from family and friends, leaving a familiar environment, decisions regarding who leaves and/or who is left behind, life threatening circumstances, experiences of persecution, violence, and loss of

Table 1
Stage of Migration Framework

Stage of Migration	Critical Variables
Pre-migration or departure	Social, political, and economic factors Separation from family and friends Decisions re: who leaves and who is left behind Leaving a familiar environment Life threatening circumstances Experiences of violence and/or persecution Loss of significant others
Transit	Perilous or safe journey of short or long duration Refugee camp or detention center stay of short or long duration Awaiting a foreign country's decision re: final relocation Loss of significant others
Resettlement	Cultural issues Reception from host country Opportunity structure of host country Discrepancy between expectations and reality Degree of cumulative stress throughout migration process

significant others are some of the issues encountered in this stage. Problems in resettlement which emerge from this phase are survivor guilt, concern for those left behind, and depression associated with the multiple losses. Post traumatic stress disorder has been reported among some whose departure experiences involved torture and violence.

PRE-MIGRATION EXPERIENCES OF SOVIET EMIGRES

Soviet Jews are the largest group of individuals leaving the Soviet Union. Anti-semitism resulting in limited social, educational, and occupational opportunities has been the primary reason for their emigration. Until recently, Soviet emigres experienced a long wait before they were able to leave their country. The long wait was a by-product of the Soviet view that emigration was considered betrayal of one's country. Thus, an application to leave involved consequences which included loss of employment, uncertainty about departure possibilities, and years of waiting while unemployed. In addition, individuals were expelled from the Communist Party and Communist Fleet, a compulsory organization for those between the ages of 14-28 (Mandel, 1990). After expulsion, former co-workers and fellow students harassed, confronted, humiliated and vilified the individual. Consent from both parents for permission to leave was also required regardless of the individual's age or nature of relationship to the parent. When parents provided consent, they too were viewed as "traitors" and they too were harassed. Some parents refused consent because it jeopardized their personal, social, and occupational lives. The issue therefore, ruptured relationships in many families (Mandel, 1990). At the point of departure and during resettlement, there has been continued concern that the decision to emigrate would further jeopardize the welfare of relatives left behind.

Prior to the recent Soviet policies of glasnost (openness) and perestroika (restructuring), emigrating individuals were not allowed to return to the Soviet Union. Thus, their departure represented a major loss–the end of contact with family and friends. The recent political changes in the Soviet Union however have relaxed Soviet emigration policies so that those presently departing are permitted to return to visit family and friends and families are permitted to leave to visit them. Thus, the degree of loss for the new arrivals has been mitigated. Moreover, many of them have had their initial application for an exit visa approved. Therefore, the years of waiting for permission to leave and the years of consequences for their emigration plans have also been reduced. These new and less severe circumstances have important implications for individual and family adaptation during the later stage of resettlement.

Although the departure circumstances for recent emigres have been changing, one segment of the new arrivals–the refusniks have had similar experiences to those of previous arrivals as they have endured years of waiting for permission to leave and years of harassment and persecution for their intent to emigrate.[2]

The following case illustration highlights the association between pre-migration experiences and issues which surface during the later phase of resettlement. A young boy's encounter with anti-

semitism in the Soviet Union and the relationship of this experience to adaptation in the United States is described.

Misha, a 13 year old boy, one of two Jewish children in his
class, had been taunted by classmates–teasing, ostracism and
verbal and physical abuse because of his Jewish background.
Although his academic performance was strong, when the
other Jewish child left the school, Misha' s functioning deteri-
orated, resulting in poor school attendance, agoraphobia and
eventually hospitalization for depression. Following hospital
discharge, he was seen by a Jewish psychiatrist recommended
by friends of his family as his parents didn't trust the state
monitored psychiatric services. He was transferred to a trade
school where he learned to repair shoes. Over time his symptoms diminished.

The child's suffering was the catalyst for the parents decision to
emigrate. After their application for an exit visa, both parents lost
their jobs and for several years were refused permission to leave
the Soviet Union. The mother was unemployed for two years. The
father eventually obtained work moonlighting in neighboring vil-
lages by installing electricity and painting homes. In 1989 (seven
years after the exit visa application), the family was permitted to
leave. However, the stresses of resettlement, the multiple un-
knowns–language, transportation, employment opportunities, the
unfamiliar environment, and the necessity to persistently interact
with strangers fostered Misha's agoraphobic difficulties expressed
in fear of leaving the home, fear of using public transportation,
fear of going to class to study English–problems which had been
associated with harassment and persecution experienced in the pre-
migration phase.

TRANSIT EXPERIENCES

In the transit phase, experiences may vary from a perilous sea
journey on a fragile boat or an illegal border crossing to an uncom-
plicated arrangement for travel on a commercial flight (Cox, 1985,

p. 74; Drachman and Ryan, 1990). It could involve years of living in limbo in a refugee camp while awaiting a final destination. It could involve a long stay in a detention center while awaiting a receiving country's decision on entry or deportation. On the other hand, an individual may leave the country of origin and within hours connect with family or friends in the new country (Drachman and Ryan, 1990).

TRANSIT EXPERIENCES OF SOVIET EMIGRES

The transit experiences of previous Soviet emigres–those who entered the United States prior to 1986 were generally orderly. Following the receipt of an exit visa, individuals departed for Vienna or Rome where they were housed in apartments while waiting for weeks to several months for their papers to be processed for final relocation. The experiences of the recent arrivals, however, have been changing. These changes are the result of complex and often conflicting forces which include foreign policy considerations, economic factors, humanitarian concerns and ethnic and minority group issues. Their influence on the experiences of recent emigres during the transit phase will be discussed below.

The entry of refugees into the United States is determined by a complex regulatory system which includes admission eligibility within the scope of an annual admission ceiling as well as an individual country ceiling (Briggs, 1984, p. 185). In accordance with the 1980 Refugee Act, a refugee must prove a well founded fear of persecution from the home country because of religion, race, nationality, membership in a particular social group or political opinion. Prior to 1986 individuals departing from the Soviet Union had little difficulty meeting the federal requirements for refugee status and the numbers leaving were so few that individuals were not constrained by the United States ceiling for that country. However, the significant rise in the Soviet emigre population eventually exhausted the admission quota for the Soviet Union. The influx of so many also raised economic concerns regarding expenditures for resettlement benefits to which refugees are entitled. The exhausted quota and the expenditures for additional refugees led to a 19%

refusal rate of Soviet Jews who applied for refugee status in 1988 (Pear, 1989b). As a result, recent emigres in Rome (the way station before final relocation) who for years had been assured entry into the United States if permitted to leave the Soviet Union, found themselves rejected by the United States and in a state of limbo.[3] Others in Moscow who were permitted by the Soviet Union to leave and who relinquished apartments, terminated employment, renounced Soviet citizenship and gave up entitlements to housing and medical care found themselves stranded in Moscow as the United States either refused the refugee status or terminated the processing of visa applications (Barringer, 1988). To deal with the crisis, the Immigration and Naturalization Service (I.N.S.) permitted some individuals to enter the country as parolees. This status created a controversy as parolees are not entitled to the resettlement services offered to refugees; they have difficulty obtaining citizenship; and those assigned to this status were required to obtain an affidavit from an American citizen pledging financial support (Gordon, 1988b).

Foreign policy issues which commonly affect the lives of immigrants and refugees have added complexity to the picture. As the political tensions between the Soviet Union and the United States have eased, it has become increasingly difficult for the United States government to continue to portray its new ally as oppressive. A debate in Congress reflects this position as some have suggested the new arrivals can no longer be conceived of as refugees under the Gorbachev policy of openness. Others have countered that glasnost has "allowed freer expression of virulent anti-semitic sentiments by grass roots organizations" (Pear, 1989b). The view that a segment of the Soviet emigre population includes economic migrants rather than refugees has also been forwarded. These arguments translate into categorizing some emigres outside of the refugee status which ultimately carry fewer benefits and services.

Israeli pressure on the United States to reject individuals who have received Israeli visas in the Soviet Union has been another political force as many have changed their destination for the United States after arriving in Rome (Rosenthal 1988; Gordon, 1988a). This pressure has been countered by humanitarian and philosophical beliefs regarding the freedom to choose one's destination (Pear, 1989b). The ethnic and minority group forces which have entered the arena revolve around the view that Soviet emigres have received preferential treatment while Latin-Americans and Asians who have been persecuted and who define themselves as refugees have been denied entry into the United States. The pressure from ethnic and minority groups intensified when the Reagan Administration increased the number of Soviets admitted as refugees by reducing the number of places reserved for Southeast Asians (Shenon, 1989; Pear, 1989a).

The forces cited above have created a state of limbo for many emigres as some have had a long wait in Rome while uncertain about their status and destination. Others have been denied entry as refugees into the United States after years of waiting for an exit visa while assured admission if permitted to leave. Others have arrived as parolees without resettlement benefits. Some families have also been separated, as members who left the Soviet Union during and after 1988 have been unable to reunify with members who arrived earlier. Some extended families who arrived together in Rome have also been separated. The separation of families is particularly problematic as the Soviet Jewish family is a tightly knit group. The closeness is reflected in common family arrangements where parents often live with their married children; they assume a major caretaking role and influence over their grandchildren; and mothers and adult daughters maintain strong ties and frequent contact.

The following case illustrates an individual's state of uncertainty and separation from family during the transit phase.

Dina, a 53 year old widow arrived in Rome with her family which was comprised of two daughters, one of whom was married and had a child. Although the entire family applied for admission into the United States, the married daughter and her family were granted entry while Dina and the other daughter remained in a long period of uncertainty while waiting for their papers to be processed for final relocation. Dina became increasingly despondent in Rome as many of her compatriots were refused entry into the United States and her uncertainty about her status and final relocation mounted. The separation from her daughter, the loss of her significant role in raising her grandchild, the years of waiting for an exit visa from the Soviet Union, and the long wait and uncertain outcome regarding her final destination culminated in severe symptoms of depression during the transit phase. Although she was eventually admitted into the United States, her adjustment in the later phase of resettlement was difficult and slow and made more complex by experiences in the transit phase.

RESETTLEMENT EXPERIENCES

As individuals resettle in the new country, cultural issues assume prominence. These issues include different views on health, mental health, education, help-seeking behavior, child rearing practices, and the degree of cultural consonance/dissonance between the country of origin and the receiving country. Cultural factors also assume prominence in the interactions between service personnel and their clients. The reception offered by the host country, the extent of services available, the degree of cumulative stress experienced by the immigrant, and the discrepancy between the individual's expectation and the quality of actual life in the United States are issues which also surface in resettlement. Depression, suicide ideation and suicide attempts, substance and chemical abuse, parent/child conflict, and wife and child abuse are among the commonly reported problems (Drachman and Ryan, 1990). As men and women shift in their traditional marital roles (particularly when wives are employed and husbands are unemployed or earn less than the wives), marital conflict or dissolution surface even among cultures where divorce is rare.

RESETTLEMENT EXPERIENCES OF SOVIET EMIGRES

For the Soviets, there have been unexpected difficulties obtaining work or resuming an occupation for which they have been trained. Many of the emigres who have been well educated have experienced lowered status as they have shifted from "Soviet engineer, teacher, musician," to "American taxi driver." Some have been unprepared for the multiple choices available to them in different aspects of U.S. life; and many have been unprepared for the absence of services such as housing, employment, occupational training, medical and dental care which have been the rights of citizens in the Soviet Union (Drachman and Ryan, 1990; Mandel, 1990).

The Soviet press reports on the United States, which often highlighted crime, homelessness and limited service entitlements, and the emigres' distrust of the Soviet government and their dismissal of Soviet claims have led many to misunderstand the degree to which social problems affect the quality of life in the United States. Thus, many emigres have been jolted by unrealistic expectations and have been unprepared for the level of struggle experienced in the new country. Some have questioned their decision to emigrate (Drachman and Ryan, 1990; Mandel, 1990).

Cultural differences have influenced service utilization and service provision. For example, voluntary service organizations and providers are foreign concepts to emigres as service personnel in the Soviet Union are government employees who are viewed as bureaucrats and are frequently manipulated by consumers in order to receive the needed service. The interactions between the emigres and United States service personnel have therefore been misunderstood as many emigres have treated service providers in a similar fashion to the Soviet "bureaucrat" and workers who have not understood this culturally normative behavior have perceived the emigres as demanding and manipulative (Mandel, 1990).

Different views on mental health also exist. Depression, for example, is perceived in the Soviet Union as a biological entity and bio-chemical treatment is offered. A refugee client experiencing depression, therefore, expects to be treated with a pill. A service provider who attempts to deal with the depression through a commonly used method of "talking therapy" is not only perceived as strange but is also viewed as incompetent as the client doesn't receive what he/she thinks is needed (Goldstein, 1984). This issue assumes greater complexity as psychiatry has been used as a form of social control in the Soviet Union; and a service provider who initiates a talking therapeutic approach is likely to be received with suspicion (Goldstein, 1984; Drachman and Ryan 1988, p. 37).

Religious beliefs and practices have also influenced service. Many of the Soviet Jewish emigres are atheists as they have been raised in an atheist culture. The different views on religious life between Soviet and American Jews have frequently been misunderstood by Soviet clients and American Jewish service providers and organizations as workers have encouraged religious activity and emigres have assumed services as conditional on religious involvement (Ryan and Drachman, 1985; Mandel, 1990).

The forces cited above often interact with one another and create a chaotic situation for an individual. The following illustration describes the situation as it has been "played out" and experienced by numerous clients. Prior to departure, a Soviet emigre is likely to hold the idea that American resources will be obtainable through one's efforts and industriousness. This view is often buttressed by letters and/or photographs from family or friends living in the United States which depict resources of a family car and new American clothing. Although social problems in the United States had been highlighted by the Soviet government, they tend to be minimized by the emigre as government statements are perceived as either untrue or exaggerated due to distrust of government claims. After arrival in the United States, the emigre encounters the costs of housing and utilities, medical and dental care and difficulty obtaining employment. The individual's basic needs press him/her to request services which have been Soviet entitlements; and the expectation of similar entitlements in the new country of rich resources appears logical. When the worker explains the limitations on United States services, the emigre assumes the worker is withholding them as this is a common experience with Soviet service personnel who are seen as bureaucrats. The assumption that services are being withheld appears validated as the individual knows compatriots in the United States who have received more services than he/she has been able to secure. When the worker explains some emigres are refugees who are entitled to more services than others who are immigrants and parolees, the individual views this as illogical as he/she views him/herself as no different from other compatriots. Moreover, the worker is often unable to explain why the emigres have different immigration statuses due to unfamiliarity with the foreign policy and economic issues, and conflicting domestic agendas which drive immigration procedures. The reactions of emigres to this situation have varied from rage, depression, unrelenting pursuit of workers and persistent demand for services, a sense of impotence resulting from the lack of control over one's life first created by the Soviet Union and now by the United States; despair over the decision to emigrate as the individual's situation is perceived as worse than before due to the added problems of losses of people and possessions, language difficulty, adjustment to a new culture and diminished hope for a better life.

IMPLICATIONS FOR SERVICE DELIVERY

The framework outlined in the discussion facilitates exploration of important areas related to the migration process which influence individual and family adaptation such as years of deprivation and persecution prior to emigration from the Soviet Union. Attention to the transit phase uncovers the experiences of separation of families and the long state of uncertainty regarding final relocation. In resettlement, when cultural issues become prominent, methods of helping may need to be altered or tailored to the cultural group. For example, interviewing with questions of a personal nature or using a "talking therapeutic" approach aimed at problem resolution should be undertaken with caution due to the cultural misunderstandings which arise from these procedures.

The significant rise in the immigrant population and its projected rise for the beginning of the 21st century implies that service personnel will be in increasing contact with immigrants both in the present and in the near future. Since the I.N.S. has a significant influence over the lives of this growing population, it is important for service personnel and organizations to understand the I.N.S. system. Familiarity with the system will facilitate an understanding of the foreign policy issues, economic factors and domestic agendas which influence its procedures and ultimately influence peoples' lives. An understanding of I.N.S. will assist worker intervention in the system so that the necessary advocacy work on behalf of individuals or populations who are disadvantaged by its procedures (such as those experienced by recent Soviet emigres) can be undertaken. Understanding and work with the I.N.S. will also facilitate helping clients negotiate the system on their own. Worker knowledge of those immigration procedures which create serious problems for people also implies there is an important role aimed at influencing immigration policy and practices.

As service personnel and organizations become involved with the I.N.S., international work is likely to evolve. For example, there is a potential function and service role for an educational program provided by United States personnel and offered in the Soviet Union which could cover the following information: differences between the two countries regarding entitlement to services; issues involved in becoming certified in the United States to practice in the different professions in which many emigres have been trained; the potential for lowered status resulting from difficulties and time entailed in re-certification which involve learning a new language, additional educational requirements and economic expenditures for the training; the phenomenon of unemployment in the United States; the cost of housing and the nature of the free market. Such a program has the potential to dispel myths about life in the United States and reduce the unrealistic expectations held by many emigres regarding their immediate future. The knowledge offered could provide individuals with an opportunity for a more informed decision on emigration and greater preparedness for experiences likely to be encountered in the new country.

Finally, there is a central role for indigenous personnel in providing services to the newly arriving groups. Their cultural and linguistic understanding is beneficial to both consumers and service providers. They possess knowledge and experience which correspond to the newcomer client thus facilitating client discussion and worker understanding of the situation; and they have the capacity to inform the professional service community on cultural issues particularly as culture relates to views on health, mental health, family, education, service provision and help-seeking behavior.

NOTES

1. The 1980 Refugee Reform Act defines a refugee as an individual who is outside of and unable or unwilling to avail him/herself of the protection of his/-her home country because of persecution or a well founded fear of persecution due to race, religion, nationality, membership in a particular social group or political opinion. In this paper, refugees and emigres are defined in accordance with the above definition. An immigrant is defined in this paper as an individual who migrates to take up residence in a new country.

2. Refusniks are individuals who attempted to emigrate but were persistently refused exit visas.

3. As of October 1, 1989, individuals from the Soviet Union seeking entry into the United States were required to apply at the American embassy in Moscow thus phasing out Rome and Vienna as future ports of entry into the United States. Presently there are about 30,000 emigres in Rome waiting for their final relocation papers to be processed. Procedures in Rome are estimated to take a year.

BIBLIOGRAPHY

Barringer, F., Ire in Moscow at Americans on visa delay. *The New York Times,* July 14, 1988, p. 9.

Briggs, V.M. (1984). *Immigration policy and the American labor force.* Baltimore, Md.: Johns Hopkins University Press.

Cox, D. (1985). Welfare services for migrants: Can they be better planned? *International Migration,* 23(1), 73-93.

Dewind, J. (1990). Haitian boat people in the United States: Background for social service providers. In D. Drachman (Ed.) *Social Services to refugee populations,* (pp. 7-56). Washington, D.C., National Institute of Mental Health.

Drachman, D. (1990). *Social services to refugee populations.* Washington, D.C., National Institute of Mental Health.

Drachman, D. and Ryan, A.S. (1990). Immigrants and refugees. In A. Gitterman (Ed.), *Handbook of social work practice with vulnerable populations.* N.Y., Columbia University Press.

Drachman, D. & Ryan, A.S. (1988). *Final report. Social work practice with refugee populations: Curriculum development in graduate social work education.* Washington, D.C., National Institute of Mental Health.

Gil, R. (1990). Cuban refugees: Implications for clinical social work practice, (pp. 7-72). In D. Drachman (Ed.) *Social services to refugee populations.* Washington, D.C., National Institute of Mental Health.

Goldstein, E. (1984). "Homo Sovieticus" in transition: Psychoanalysis and problems of social adjustment. *Journal of the American Academy of Psychoanalysis,* 12(1), 115-126.

Gordon, M. (1988a). Exit for Soviet Jews, conflict for Americans. *The New York Times*, Aug. 14, 1988. Section 4, p. 2.

Gordon, M. (1988b). U.S. to ease backlog in Soviet emigration but draws criticism. *The New York Times*, Dec. 9, 1988, p. 1.

Johnston, W. & Packer, A. (1988). *Workplace 2000: Work and workers for the twenty-first century*. Indianapolis: Hudson Institute.

Keller, S. (1975). *Uprooting and social change: the role of refugees in development*. Delhi: Manohar Book Service.

Mandel, L. (1990). Soviet refugees. In D. Drachman (Ed.) *Social services to refugee populations*, (pp. 73-90). Washington, D.C., National Institute of Mental Health.

Meyer, C. (1984). Working with new immigrants. *Social Work*, 29(2), 99.

O, S.L. & Porr, P. (1990). Social work practice with Indochinese refugees. In D. Drachman (Ed.) (pp. 91-121). *Social services to refugee populations*. Washington, D.C., National Institute of Mental Health.

Pear, R. (1989a). U.S. raises quota of Soviet refugees by cutting Asians. *The New York Times*. Jan. 12, 1989, p. 1.

Pear, R. (1989b). U.S. drafts plans to curb admission of Soviet Jews. *The New York Times*, Sept. 3, 1989.

Rosenthal, A.M. Justice at State. *The New York Times*, July 12, 1988, p. 25.

Ryan, A.S. and Drachman, D. (1985). *Final report: Mental health/crisis intervention training for refugee resettlement workers*. Washington, D.C., Office of Refugee Resettlement, Department of Health and Human Services.

Saperia, P.A. & Stolow, D., Oct. 24, 1989. Changes in U.S. Consular practices in Moscow: Fact sheet. Hebrew Immigrant Aid Society.

Shenon, P. (1989). U.S. proposes rise of up to 150,000 in new refugees. *The New York Times*, April 6, 1989, p. 1.

Stein, B. (1986). The experience of being a refugee: Insights from the literature. In C. Williams and J. Westermeyer (Eds.), *Refugee mental health in resettlement countries*, (pp. 5-23). Washington, D.C.: Hemisphere Publishing.

U.S. Bureau of the Census. U.S. Census of Population, 1970. Final Report, PC(1)-C1.

U.S. Bureau of the Census. U.S. Census of Population, 1980. Final Report P.C. 80(1)-C1.

Wall Street Journal, Dec. 13, 1989, p. 10.

Training for Cross-Cultural Social Work with Immigrants, Refugees, and Minorities: A Course Model

Carole Pigler Christensen

SUMMARY. This paper describes the development, format, and procedures of a course designed to prepare social work students to work with immigrants, refugees, and minorities. Historical, sociopolitical, economic, and psychosocial factors are considered. The model emphasizes experiential learning in classroom and community settings, which enables students to integrate theory and skills related to practice. Emphasis is placed on the development of self-awareness as a major aspect of training.

From earliest times, North American societies have been pluralistic, composed first of indigenous peoples, and later of European and Black cultural and racial groups (Anderson and Frideres, 1981; Mindel and Habenstein, 1981). In recent years, immigrants and refugees from the Caribbean, Asia, Africa, and Latin America have arrived in significant numbers, expanding the multicultural nature of Canada and of the United States. Consequently, social work educators are challenged to prepare students to work effectively with clients from widely diverse ethnic, cultural, and racial (ECR) backgrounds. A review of the literature suggests that educators and practitioners are often overwhelmed by the call to respond sensitively to a multitude of life-experiences, values, and family patterns

Carole Pigler Christensen, MSW, DEd, is Director and Professor, University of British Columbia, School of Social Work. Mailing Address: School of Social Work, 6201 Cecil Green Park Road, Vancouver, B.C. V6T 1W5.

(Dana, 1981; Multicultural Workers' Network, 1981; Devore and Schlesinger, 1981). The need to develop innovative teaching models to enhance cross-cultural awareness, knowledge, and practice skills is widely acknowledged, (Christensen, 1984; White, 1982). This paper describes an original model for teaching cross-cultural social work, developed by the author over a fifteen year period. Its purpose is to offer a unique approach, which emphasizes innovative experiential teaching methods and assignments, readily adaptable to other pluralistic locales.

SOCIAL WORK'S RESPONSE TO PLURALISM

Like the United States, Canada is often referred to as ''a country of immigrants.'' Although officially considered a bilingual country having ''two founding nations,'' the French and the British, immigrants of other backgrounds comprise one-third of the population (Kallen, 1982). The most preferred immigrants and refugees were traditionally from Western and Northern European countries but, a combination of manpower needs and international migration pressures led to an influx, first of eastern and southern Europeans and, more recently, of Third World migrants (Christensen, 1986a). Following the adoption of ''non-racist'' immigration regulations in the 1960s, the ''point-system'' emphasized education and job-related skills for those seeking landed immigrants status (Hawkins, 1972). About 17% of all immigrants are admitted as refugees (Canadian Task Force on Mental Health Issues Affecting Immigrants and Refugees, 1988). The total non-White population in Canada, called ''visible minorities,'' is approximately 5.6% (Statistics Canada, 1989a), but in cities such as Toronto, Montreal, Halifax, Vancouver, and Calgary, percentages are estimated to be 6-10%. Thousands of illegal immigrants are believed to be in Canada (Robinson, 1983). The highest number of recent immigrants and refugees (70%) have been from the Third World (Statistics Canada, 1989b), a percentage expected to remain constant through the year 2001 (Samuel, 1988). Unlike the melting pot philosophy adopted by the United States, Canada officially adopted a multicultural policy in 1971, and is popularly called a "mosaic," in which immigrant groups are allowed to maintain their heritage and cultures.

The social work profession has not adequately reflected the multicultural and multiracial nature of Canadian society, either in manpower or in training programs (Christensen, 1986b; Yelaja, 1990). Although the policy statement of the Canadian Association of Schools of Social Work encourages the adoption of content "relevant to the constituencies that we aim to serve," specific, enforceable guidelines are only now being considered (Canadian Association of Schools of Social Work, 1991). Although in place in the United States for some time now, equal opportunity employment policies and student admissions procedures for minorities have only recently come into being in some Canadian universities.

BACKGROUND AND RATIONALE

In 1974, a one-semester (13 week) undergraduate elective was initiated in a Social Work program at a Canadian anglophone University in Montreal, Quebec–a metropolis where the majority of the population is francophone; 11% are anglophone; and 16% are immigrants, most of whom are of neither British nor French background. Many speak neither English nor French (Statistics Canada, 1989b).

The course was initially entitled "Minority Groups and Social Welfare." Notably, the author designed the course in response to minority students' requests that more attention be given to sociopolitical as well as psychosocial factors affecting immigrant and minority clients. Initially, the course focused on how immigration regulations, and formal and informal social welfare and social service policies, affect immigrants, refugees, and minority populations. As the course evolved, emphasis was increasingly placed on experiential components, in response to students' need to develop skills directly related to practice. The course title was changed to "Cross-Cultural Perspectives in Social Work Practice," and later, to the present title, "Social Work Practice in a Multicultural Context." The course description reads:

Preparation for work with a multicultural and multiracial clientele, including immigrants and refugees. Topics include the impact of formal and informal social policies and institutions on the well-being of immigrants and minorities. The relationship between culture and social work practice is explored. Opportunities for experiential learning in classroom and community settings allow students to interact with selected cultural groups.

Students represent an increasingly wide range of immigrant backgrounds. Most have parents or grandparents who were immigrants or refugees, and many were born in other countries. Currently, approximately one-third are Canadians of British background; one-third are Jewish; one-quarter are Italian, and the remainder are commonly of Greek, Portuguese, Eastern European, Caribbean or Canadian-born Black, or Asian (Chinese, Japanese, East Indian) background. Usually, one or two are aboriginals (Native Canadians) and an equal number are on foreign student visas. Students thus have opportunities to learn from classmates who are living the immigrant experience.

COURSE OBJECTIVES, OUTLINES, AND PROCEDURES

The objectives of the course are to:

1. provide a conceptual framework for the analysis of current policies and practices affecting immigrants, refugees and minorities, in historical perspective;
2. increase awareness of the meaning of one's culture, ethnicity, and race when relating to clients from backgrounds other than one's own;
3. increase knowledge and understanding of similarities and differences manifested in individuals and groups, through readings and direct contact with selected communities;
4. develop beginning analytical and assessment skills which acknowledge the contributions of ethnicity, culture, and race as factors in the etiology of client problems;

5. encourage the critical evaluation of social work values, theories, methods, and policies, as they affect immigrants, refugees, and others from ethnic, cultural, and racial groups encountered in practice.

The 3-credit course (consisting of 2 hours of class time and one hour out-of-class time) is divided into two major parts. During the first 6 weeks, emphasis is placed on: (a) experiential exercises with the aim of establishing an atmosphere of trust and openness; (b) a theoretical framework, including major concepts and relevant terminology; (c) growth in awareness of self and others, by experiencing a cross-cultural relationship. The last 6 weeks offer an opportunity to meet informally with people from selected immigrant or minority communities. The literature suggests that having a professor from an immigrant or minority background (which is true in this case) may offer students an additional opportunity to confront personal and societal issues relating to ethnicity, culture, and race (Mizio & Delany, 1981).

Session 1

Students are asked to sit in a circle, facing each other, for the duration of the course. In keeping with the aim of having students begin to share attitudes, feelings, and experiences, the initial class begins with an experiential exercise.

Experiential Exercise

Students are asked to respond to the following questions, used to introduce class members to each other:

1. Your name.
2. What is your ECR background?
3. How do others become aware of your ECR background?
4. How important is your ECR background in your daily life?
5. What do you hope to gain from taking this course?

Each student chooses someone s/he does not know well with whom to share responses. This places them in a situation similar to that of a client and worker who are likely to be uncomfortable, initially, discussing such topics. Fifteen minutes are allotted. Students then introduce their partners, summarizing what they have learned.

In response to question 3, visible minority students, whether immigrants or not, mention color as the variable that inevitably distinguishes them from majority group White Canadians. Many note that in Canada, to be non-White is to be considered "ethnic," which carries negative connotations. Other factors mentioned as indicators of ECR identity include accented speech, last names, and mode of dress. Students saying that people are aware of their ECR background only if they choose to tell them invariably appear to be White, with British or French last names. Often, they are of "mixed" ancestry. For example, one student introduced to the class as being of French-Canadian and East Indian background said:

> People assume I'm French-Canadian because of my last name. Most of the time, I don't bother to say that my mother is Indian. When I do, the reaction is usually one of surprise, and may even be negative.

Question 4, "How important is your ECR background to you?" draws responses from "not at all important" to "always very important." Positive comments often indicate a sense of pride, instilled in the country of origin, or in an "ethnic" neighborhood in Canada. For example, Italian students often attend public schools where the principal, teachers, and most students are Italian immigrants. On the other hand, second or third generation visible minority students often note that pride in their Canadian identity is hampered, since their hyphenated identity is not always maintained by choice. A third generation Chinese-Canadian student commented:

> Everyone asks if I'm from Hong Kong, China, or Japan. It annoys me that no one seems to expect me to be just plain Canadian, even though I have no accent.

A Black student remarked:

> I'm a sixth generation Black Canadian from Nova Scotia. I'm tired of being asked where I come from by white immigrants.

Usually, at least one majority group (British or French) student admits that being part of this group brings privileges in the form of psychological well-being, social acceptance, or more tangible advantages (e.g., "We lived in better areas of the city than those occupied by most immigrant groups."). The discussion helps students begin to acknowledge feelings attached to immigrant status and ECR identity.

In discussing their personal objectives when choosing this elective (Question 5), most students express an interest in increasing their understanding of various groups, to work with them more effectively. A minority of the students usually admit to hoping to rid themselves of biases about various groups. Others may wish to understand reasons for aspects of their societal status, as immigrants or ECR minorities.

The course outline and requirements are then introduced, emphasizing that the theoretical framework may be applied to any immigrant or ECR group, and to any multicultural or multiracial context. The first concepts discussed are those in the course title, "Social Work Practice in a Multicultural Context." Students are encouraged to critically examine several classic definitions of *Social Work*, including the following:

> A professional service, based upon scientific knowledge and skill in human relations, which assists individuals, alone or in groups, to obtain social and person satisfaction and independence. (Freidlander, 1968, p. 4)

Discussion of old and new definitions allows students to become aware of the cultural basis (i.e., Western, North-American, White, and middle class) of professional Social Work, which values "scientific" knowledge, independence, and personal, rather than collective, satisfaction. Students note that socioeconomic class, ethnicity, culture, race and immigrant or refugee status are not generally mentioned in definitions.

Culture is defined as consisting of commonalities around which people have developed values, norms, family styles, social roles, and behaviors, in response to the historical, political, economic, and social realities they face (Pinderhughes, 1984). Therefore, immigrants and refugees' cultures represent more than traditions and folk-ways; they are not static, but change due to the North American experience. *Cross-cultural social work* is defined as any encounter in which the worker and client come from different ECR backgrounds. *Multicultural contexts* exist wherever people from a number of ECR groups are in daily interaction. It is noted that class, race, and ethnicity are often closely associated, and that race is often confused with culture.

Assignment 1

During Session I, census figures for Montreal are placed on the blackboard and the class chooses, by majority vote, three ECR groups for study during the second half of the course. The immigrant groups chosen have included (in order of popularity of choice): Blacks, Jews, Chinese, Italians, Vietnamese, Greeks, Latin Americans, Japanese, South Asians (East Indians, Pakistanis); aboriginal Canadians are also a popular choice. Students divide into three study groups, of approximately equal size, respecting individual interests. Lots are drawn to determine which group will present first. The instructions for this assignment read:

> Invite persons from selected ethnic, cultural, or racial groups to share their viewpoints, perceptions, and experiences highlighting material of relevance to social workers, such as immigrant adjustment; life-style; child rearing and family practices; and experience of minority status. During the following week, students are to prepare, for class presentation, an analysis of what was heard and experienced, integrating concepts and theories. Grading is based on the degree to which students integrate learning in a clear and useful manner. This assignment is worth 35% of the final grade.

Each student receives the same group grade, to sensitize students to the immigrant and minority person's experience of being "in the same boat" with an identifiable group, and judged accordingly. Group members soon become aware of the contributions and liabilities of those with whom they are arbitrarily linked and are able to note responses and group dynamics.

Experience with this assignment has led to the stipulations that students: (1) do not choose their own immigrant or minority group (the level of emotional involvement may hamper an honest and objective examination of the group); (2) avoid inviting designated immigrant or minority "spokespersons" (some use the classroom to promote a particular view of their group); (3) invite males and females from a variety of age groups and life-situations. The groups use the ensuing weeks working on Assignment 1, which is actually presented during the last six weeks of the course.

Knowledge and skills gained this session: Knowledge of different groups' feelings about their ECR or immigrant status; increased comfort and self-awareness.

Session II

A major focus of this session is on raising students' sensitivity to how we learn cultural values, and on becoming aware of their underlying emotional components. The transmission and practice implications of social work values are also considered.

Experiential Exercise

1. List six (6) values passed on to you by parents or caregivers.
2. How did your parents or caregivers make you aware of important values?
3. Circle the values that you consider to be peculiar to your cultural, ethnic, or racial group.
4. Place a "✓" next to the values that you still adhere to, and an "X" next to those that you no longer adhere to.

Students divide into groups of three to discuss responses. Most are surprised that certain values are generally held in common, including the importance of the family, honesty, hard work, education, and equality or fair play. Differences in interpretation of the meaning of these values, in behavioral terms, evokes lively discussion and debate. The danger of inadvertently imposing one's own value system is about always identified. Students become aware that most values are passed on by example and by non-verbal means. They also gain insights about how, and why, the values of immigrants change over time, and the effects this has on intergenerational relations.

For the purposes of this course, the majority group is defined as having most of the power, privilege, and prestige within a given society (Kallen, 1982). It is the group from which the elite classes and decision-makers are primarily drawn, and whose culture and history are transmitted and sanctioned by major societal institutions (e.g., government bodies, the media, and schools). This group determines immigration and refugee policies. The opposite is true of minority groups, who are subjectively aware of unequal treatment due to physical, social, or cultural characteristics. In Canada, immigrants and refugees who are of neither British nor French ancestry become part of a minority group.

Assignment 2

The log is introduced by asking each student to find someone (not a client) of a different ECR background than him/herself who will agree to meet weekly, for about 50 minutes, for the next 6-8 weeks, in an informal setting. The purpose is to monitor internal responses and more overt behaviors, and increase comfort when interacting with someone different from oneself. It offers an opportunity to explore topics that are taboo, including feelings about one's immigrant or ECR status; personal experiences of stereotypes, racism, prejudice, and discrimination; and viewpoints about public policies such as immigration and refugee laws, multiculturalism, and human rights legislation. Although students expect difficulty finding a willing participant, immigrants and minorities are usually pleased that social work students are interested in their views and experiences to enhance their understanding. This assignment helps to develop social work skills, including: raising and phrasing appropriate questions about the immigrant or minority persons' experience; using allotted time to gain insight into an individual's views and feelings about sensitive issues; increased empathic understanding toward a dissimilar group; active listening; and integrating theory and concepts through analysis of material presented in sessions.

The second period of this session involves a consideration of policies, terminology, and concepts from readings, including: human rights; enslavement (i.e., of Blacks in Canada); entrance status; majority group; social roles; immigrant adaptation stages; achieved and ascribed statuses; social stratification; relative deprivation, and the Vertical Mosaic. The Vertical Mosaic (Porter, 1965) suggests that Canadian immigrant groups form a hierarchy along ethnic and racial lines, with British immigrants comprising the largest elite class at the top; French Canadians and European immigrants occupying the middle ranks, along with Asians and some other non-whites; and most Blacks, and aboriginal groups on the bottom.

Knowledge and skills gained this session: Enhanced knowledge of value similarities and differences, and awareness of how immigrants change over time.

Session III

The experiential exercise introduced is designed to develop beginning awareness of how we learn to classify people, and to raise levels of consciousness about the possible consequences of such categorizations.

Experiential Exercise

Each student lists the categories of people that they think of as ''we'' and as ''they.'' Fifteen minutes are allotted to compare lists in groups of three, and a reporter is chosen to summarize the experience for the class. Students, often reluctantly, note that most of us classify ourselves and others into ''we/they'' groups, usually based on ECR identity, national origin, religion, language, class, and sex; and that initial categorizations are based on visible clues (e.g., skin color, physical features, dress), and audible (e.g., accents, verbal skills) clues. A student of Greek immigrant parents shared the following experience:

> I'll never forget when I was 5 years old, and my friend said that her parents didn't allow Greeks in the house, but she could play with me outside.

Students discuss the categorizations built into formal and informal social agency policies, such as intake, and whether one's "professional self" can avoid emotional responses that would occur in non-professional interactions.

Theories and concepts discussed pertain to the distinction between an immigrant or minority person's ethnic group identity, and the ethnic category s/he may be placed in by the dominant culture. The impact and purpose of such categorizations is considered.

Knowledge and skills gained this session: Increased self-awareness; how distinctions may lead to discriminatory behavior.

Session IV

This session begins with an experiential exercise adapted from Pinderhughes (1979).

Experiential Exercise

1. What is your ECR background?
2. What ethnic, cultural, and racial groups resided in the neighborhood where you grew up?
3. How did your family see itself as like, or different from, other groups?
4. What are your earliest images of people's color as a factor in your community?
5. How are your feelings about your ECR background influenced by the power relationships between your own group and other groups?

Students divide into groups of 4 to discuss their responses. The aim of the exercise is to help students consider power relationships among groups and their implications in society generally, and in cross-cultural social work encounters in particular. Students usually answer questions 1-3 with little difficulty, but levels of embarrassment, anger, anxiety, sadness, and guilt are raised in response to questions 4 and 5. Examples of students' comments are:

I used to wish I was not Vietnamese. Students made us use another door to enter and leave the school. But at least the teachers considered us well-behaved and good at math.

As a child, I was more attached to my West Indian nanny than to my mother. I think she was fired because my parents began to realize this too.

This class has given me my first opportunity to hear what gentiles might really think about Jews and the Holocaust. I've gotten a lot off my chest. All non-Jews don't always feel as I thought.

Group dynamics often evoke heated discussion as levels of openness and trust increase and experiences are related to theoretical concepts such as social distance, boundaries, labelling, racism, and institutionalized racism. A spokesperson summarizes each small group's experience for the class.

Knowledge and skills gained this session: Understanding of how ECR enhances or hinders life-chances where discrimination and racism are institutionalized; empathy and listening skills; dealing with feelings of self and others.

Session V

Session V introduces students to methods of control and domination used by majority groups to maintain the status quo, including: control of immigration; persecution and extermination; control of land ownership; denial of employment, wages, and advancement; separate or unequal education; denial of accommodation and use of recreational facilities; denial of the vote; perpetuation of myths and stereotypes through written and visual media; bias or omission in historical accounts; separation and segregation; denial of participation in the political and financial arenas; denial of full participation in decision-making; sanctioning of unequal expectations; control of information. That these methods and techniques are used differentially toward various groups helps to explain why some immigrant and minority groups become upwardly mobile within one or two generations, while others do not. There is often denial that such methods may be used deliberately by those in power. Majority group students find classmates may associate them with oppressive forces. Students need considerable help to deal with feelings and class dynamics. For most non-immigrant White students, hearing others' stereotypes and negative comments about their reference group is a new experience. One English-Canadian student remarked:

> It's as if Whites are the sources of all the worlds' evils, but it can be pretty hard for us too. At my summer job, the boss told us not to hire Chinese or Black immigrants. I'm not prejudiced, but what could I do? I needed the job.

Experiential Exercise

To raise awareness of how immigrants and minorities may respond to their plight, students are introduced to a concept of minority identity (Atkinson, Morten, and Sue, 1983) which proposes a five stage process: conformity; dissonance; resistance and immersion; introspection; synergetic articulation and awareness. Each stage is accompanied by different attitudes toward self; others of the same minority; others of different minority; and the dominant group. Students are asked to estimate where they (or someone they know) are on the model. This is a private exercise, due to the possibly threatening revelations that ensue. Students discuss implications of the model for social work practice. Subjective feelings that immigrants, refugees and minorities may experience, such as hopelessness, anger, frustration, powerlessness, low self-esteem, despair, rejection, and marginality are acknowledged.

Knowledge and skills gained this session: Awareness that personality development and social adjustment of immigrants and minorities differs from that of majority group individuals. Understanding of biculturality.

Session VI

Students are introduced to several styles of intergroup relations, including colonialism, neo-colonialism, dominant conformity, cultural pluralism, the melting pot, and multiculturalism (Kallen, 1982). Students consider the pros and cons, and implicit assumptions, underlying each form of intergroup relations. In preparation for this class, reading is about change strategies and methods used by immigrants, refugees, ECR groups, and mainstream institutions to improve the situation of various groups, including: information; education; lobbying; self-help; media; community development and control; institutional completeness; compensation; planning by "experts"; advocacy; confrontation; affirmative action; and innovation. Discussion centers around the effectiveness of models and remedies currently in use.

Experiential Exercise

Students are asked to examine their fieldwork placements by responding to the following questions:

1. What immigrant or ECR groups are found in the surrounding community?
2. To what extent is each of these groups represented as: voluntary and involuntary clients; professional/clerical staff; administrators; agency board members; participants in self-help or grass-roots efforts?
3. What are the implications of responses to (1) and (2) above in relation to the concepts and theories studied?
4. What change strategies and methods would you suggest to remedy the situation, and why might they be effective or ineffective?

Based on the above observations, students discuss, in groups of five, the costs and benefits of occupying a minority or majority group status in present-day Canada.

Knowledge and experience gained for this session: Increased understanding of how the experiences of immigrant and minority groups may be expressed in individual, family, and community problems, often leading to use of social services. Effects of power and control mechanism in social work and social welfare institutions; how to effect change.

Session VII

A 2-hour quiz during Session VII is mainly a test of factual knowledge. This is especially important because historical and current information about immigrants, refugees, and minorities is seldom part of the public school or university curriculum.

Part II of Course (Sessions VIII-XVIII)

The last six weeks of the course are devoted to informal discussions with guests from the three groups chosen by the students at the beginning of the term. Students will have selected people from various communities to share relevant experiences with the class (see Assignment 1 description, page 92).

To create an informal atmosphere, a lounge is used. Students often bring news clippings, books, cultural artifacts and food of the group being studied (a small budget is available). The student group responsible is expected to ensure that the 2-hour time-period is used to full advantage, allowing time for questions.

It is difficult to describe the excitement and enthusiasm when guests arrive. Through interaction with people from various groups, many students begin to realize similarities between the adjustment process, life experience, and feelings of their own group and that of immigrants and minorities with whom they believed they had little, or nothing, in common.

For the following week's analysis, students often use audio-visual aids, role-play, and games, as well as traditional didactic formats to engage the class in a discussion of what was said and understood about the guests' experiences. Class participation is usually extremely high.

Knowledge and skills gained during these sessions: Knowledge about life experiences of members of specific immigrant, refugee, and minority populations. Ability to critically examine these experiences and relate them to theoretical material.

COURSE EVALUATION AND EFFECTIVENESS

Efforts to incorporate cross-cultural learning into the social work curriculum are not always evaluated or reported. Both qualitative and quantitative methods have been used to evaluate this course. A thorough evaluation was carried out in 1977 by a specialist from the University Center for Teaching and Learning who attended and videotaped all classes. Periodically, students were also asked to fill out questionnaires, and to give written comments. Feed-back was very positive, and indicated no major changes were deemed necessary. Quantitative measures used indicated that the course was evaluated as excellent by 80% of the students and as very good by 20%. Eighty-five per cent of those enrolled evaluated the course very highly in terms of the usefulness of teaching methods, relevance to practice, ability of instructor, values clarification, and new knowledge and skills. The same percentage indicated that the objectives of the course were being met. Also, at the beginning of each term, the instructor asks students to complete a form indicating what prompted them to take the course, and what they hope to gain thereby. At the end of the term, the overwhelming majority of students indicate that they have achieved most of their goals in terms of increased self-awareness, knowledge, and skill.

Students evaluate the course anonymously on a yearly basis, using a standard Likert-type questionnaire used in all of the School's courses. Evaluations on a five-point scale (1 = strongly disagree, 5 = strongly agree) consistently average about 4.5, indicating that the course is meeting objectives, levels of learning are high, and that the instructor and teaching methods are considered effective. A large number of graduates report, years later, that they continue to use what they learned.

CONCLUSION

This paper has presented a model to prepare social work students to work with immigrants, refugees, and minorities in a multicultural and multiracial environment. The major strengths of this model are that it provides opportunities to incorporate knowledge and skills relevant to social work practice through experiential learning, enabling students to move quickly from a cognitive to a feeling level. Self-awareness is enhanced as students interact with immigrant and minority communities in class and community settings. To maintain and reinforce learning, all components of social work education, must prepare students for the realities of multicultural and multiracial societies. At a time when international migration is increasing and is expected to continue, this model is offered to help educators to meet this challenge.

REFERENCES

Anderson, Alan B., & Frideres, James S. (1981). *Ethnicity in Canada: Theoretical perspectives.* Toronto: Butterworth and Co., 1981.

Atkinson, D.R., Morten, G., & Sue, D.W. (Eds.) (1983). "Proposed minority identity development model." In *Counseling American Minorities* (pp. 191-200) Iowa: Wm. C. Brown Company Publishers.

Berry, J.W., Kalin, R., & Taylor, D.. (1977). *Multiculturalism and Ethnic Attitudes in Canada.* Ottawa: Supply and Services Canada.

Canadian Association of Schools of Social Work (1991). *Social Work Education at the Crossroads: The Challenge of Diversity. Report of the Task Force on Multicultural and Multiracial Issues in Social Work Education.* Ottawa: Canadian Association of Schools of Social Work.

Canadian Task Force on Mental Health Issues Affecting Immigrants and Refugees (1988). *After the Door Has Been Opened.* Ottawa: Health and Welfare Canada.

Christensen, C.P. (1984). Effects of Cross-Cultural training on counselor response. *Counselor Education and Supervision, 23*, 4, 311-320.

Christensen, C.P. (1986a). Minorities in Canada: Immigrant Groups. Turner, J.C., & F.J. Turner (Eds.) *Canadian Social Welfare.* Toronto: Collier MacMillan.

Christensen, C.P. (1986b). Cross-Cultural Social Work: Fallacies fears, and failings. *Intervention*, 6-15.

Christensen, C.P. (1990). Toward a Framework for Social Work Education in a Multicultural and Multiracial Canada. In Yelaja, S. *Proceedings of the Settlement and integration of new immigrants to Canada Conference*, February 17-19, 1988. Ontario: Faculty of Social Work and Centre for Social Welfare Studies, Wilfred Laurier University.

Dana, R.N. (1981). *Human Services for Cultural Minorities.* Baltimore: University Park Press.

Devore, W., & Schlesinger, E.G. (1981). *Ethnic-Sensitive Social Work Practice.* St. Lewis: The C.V. Mosby Company.

Freidlander, W.A. (1968) (3rd Edition). *Introduction to Social Welfare.* Englewood Cliffs, N.J.: Prentice Hall.

Hawkins, F. (1972). *Canada and Immigration: Public policy and public concern.* Montreal: McGill-Queen's University Press.

Kallen, E. (1982). *Ethnicity and Human Rights in Canada.* (Toronto: Gage Publishing Ltd.).

Mindel, C.H., & Habenstein, R.W. (1981). *Ethnic Families in America, Patterns and Variations.* (2nd Edition). New York: Elsevier North Holland Inc.

Mizio, E., & Delaney, A. (1981). *Training for Service Delivery to Minority Clients.* New York: Family Service Association of America.

Multicultural Worker's Network (1981). *The Family: Interventive Strategies in a Multicultural Context.* Conference Proceedings, Toronto, Ontario.

Pinderhughes, E.B. (1979). Teaching Empathy in Cross-Cultural Social Work. *Social Work,* 312-318.

Pinderhughes, E.B. (1984). The Significance of Power in Human Behaviour: Proposal for Adding Ethnic Minority Content to the Human Behaviour Curriculum. C. Jacobs, Ed. *Ethnic Minority Content in Social Work Education.* Smith College School of Social Work.

Porter, J. (1965) *The Vertical Mosaic.* Toronto: University of Toronto Press.

Robinson, W.G. (1983). *Illegal Immigrants in Canada: A report to the Honourable Lloyd Axworthy, Minister of Employment and Immigration.* Ottawa: Minister of Supply and Services Canada.

Samuel, J.T. (1988). Immigration and Visible minorities in the year 2001: A projection, *Canadian Ethnic Studies, XX,* 2, 92-100.

Statistics Canada (1989a). Census of Canada. Ottawa: Ministry of Supply and Services Canada.

Statistics Canada (1989b). Dimensions: Profile of the immigrant population. Ottawa: Ministry of Supply and Services Canada.

White, B.W. (Ed.) (1982). *Color in a White Society.* Silver Spring, Maryland: National Association of Social Workers, Inc.

Yelaja, S. (1990). *Proceedings of the Settlement and integration of new immigrants to Canada Conference,* February 17-19, 1988. Ontario: Faculty of Social Work and Centre for Social Welfare Studies, Wilfred Laurier University.

Paraprofessionals in Refugee Resettlement

Joann Ivry

SUMMARY. The increased demands of refugee resettlement have directed attention to the role and function of indigenous paraprofessionals, who share a common background and experience with the client population. With training and supervision, such paraprofessionals can bridge cultural and linguistic barriers, and serve as role models. This article examines this topic from the experience of the recent Soviet Jewish refugee resettlement program in Boston.

INTRODUCTION

Refugees services in the United States consist of a complex interlocking web of public and private institutions and programs. In general, the federal government establishes the legal parameters, policies and procedures for refugee immigration, and allocates resources to state and local governments for refugee cash assistance and medicaid programs. The government also establishes programmatic guidelines for resettlement services and allocates funds to nine officially recognized private voluntary agencies which organize, coordinate and administer the refugee program in the United States. These voluntary migration agencies are part of an association known as the American Council of Voluntary Agencies, referred to colloquially as the "Volags," which in conjunction with a national network of affiliated sponsors, implement the refugee program (Brown, 1982). The Volags have historically

Joann Ivry, PhD, is Assistant Professor, Hunter College School of Social Work, 129 E. 79th Street, New York, NY 10021. This paper is dedicated to the New American staff of Boston Jewish Family and Children's Service.

99

played a critical role in refugee resettlement, being responsible for the organization and coordination of an international migration service which handles reception and resettlement of refugees in the United States from many countries of the world, particularly Europe, Cuba, Haiti, Southeast Asia, and what used to be called the Soviet Union.

Despite the establishment of core services to which all refugees are entitled, refugee resettlement services in the United States remain characterized by diversity rather than by a "single, logically consistent effort" (Haines, 1985, p. 7). For example, while all the Volags must arrange that each refugee entering the states has a sponsor, there is considerable diversity in the type of sponsors used. These may be "individual or group sponsors, agencies or institutional sponsors, or congregational sponsors" (Schwamm, Greenstone and Hoffman, 1982, p. 26). According to Rubin (1982), there are essentially two models of refugee resettlement. The first, family sponsorship, relies primarily on local families which sponsor refugees often in association with community churches, and are loosely connected with the national Volag which recruited them. In the family sponsorship model, services are usually provided on a voluntary basis without the involvement of professional social workers, at least, not in the initial phases of resettlement. In the second model, defined as community sponsorship, volunteerism is ancillary, and "central to this service model is an agency which represents the community and assumes sponsorship for the resettlement of the family" (Rubin, 1982, p. 302).

The Hebrew Immigrant Aid Society (known as HIAS), one of the nine recognized Volags, is a world-wide Jewish refugee organization and has been an active participant in refugee services for over one hundred years. HIAS's primary responsibility is to assist refugees in transit by providing them with financial assistance, migration counseling and assistance in preparation of documents to ensure entrance into the United States. While the refugees are awaiting approval of their emigration papers, HIAS, in consultation with the refugees, assigns them to a host community in the United States. This assignment is usually done on the basis of family reunion, job opportunities and the number of refugees each community is able to assist. HIAS's responsibility for refugees terminates once they arrive in the sponsoring community. At that point the local Jewish family service agency, in collaboration with other Jewish communal service agencies, assumes responsibility for the refugee and provides a range of resettlement services including orientation, financial assistance, housing, health care, language classes, job placement, and counseling. By and large, HIAS and its network of affiliate Jewish family service agencies have utilized the community sponsorship model of resettlement services and generally have relied on professional social workers to be the primary service providers. Within the community sponsorship model, diversity also exists in the use of professional and paraprofessional staff. This paper will examine the emergence of the role and function of paraprofessionals in the resettlement of Soviet Jewish refugees.

AGENCY-REFUGEE ENCOUNTER

Soviet Jews began their exodus from the then Soviet Union in the early 1970's, with the majority going to Israel. In the mid-1970's a shift in the migration pattern occurred, with the majority of emigrants choosing to enter the United States. Between 1975 and 1980, 90,000 Soviet Jews entered the United States as refugees (Simon, 1985, p. 181). In 1980, the numbers of Soviet Jews allowed to leave the Soviet Union was drastically reduced as a result of deteriorating international relations and the Soviet invasion of Afghanistan. However, with perestroika and glasnost, the situation was reversed in the late 1980's and Soviet Jews once again began exiting from the Soviet Union. Between 1986 and 1989, "the number of Jews permitted to leave the Soviet Union jumped from 900 to 8,000 to 21,000 . . ." and it was projected that in 1990 40,000 Soviet-Jewish refugees would be resettled in the United States (Zukerman, 1990, pp. 100 & 101). Faced with this huge influx of refugees over the past twenty years, the Jewish communal system had "to adapt and develop programs for the new Soviet client" (Gilson, 1976, p. 7).

The new Soviet Jewish client is quite unlike his forebears who emigrated in large numbers to the United States in the first quarter of the twentieth century. In contrast to the earlier waves of Russian Jewish immigrants, who were religiously or culturally identified Jews but poor, rural and largely unprofessional, the recent arrivals as described by Gold are "educated, skilled and possess extensive urban experience, have little religious training . . . or experience with voluntary association . . ." (as quoted by Showstack, 1989, p. 66). Similar to their forebears, however, the recent wave of Soviet Jewish refugees is also fleeing religious and ethnic persecution, despite hopes that communism would create a new social order free of ethnic hatred and prejudice (Simon, 1985).

Though victims of discrimination, Jews from the former Soviet Union have been molded by the Soviet political and economic authoritarian system (Freedman, 1977). Neither allowed to live as Jews nor to integrate fully into Soviet society, Soviet Jews represent "a curious mixture of Soviet acculturation and Jewish history" (Schwamm et al., 1982, p. 27). It is this last point particularly that is critical to understand the encounter between Soviet Jewish refugee clients and the professional social worker in the Jewish family service agency.

From the very first years of this encounter, mutual criticisms and frustrations were often expressed. As Brodsky wrote in 1982, social workers despaired that they would be able to work or establish relationships with this population, and noted that the Russian clients were ". . . unresponsive, overly suspicious and withdrawn" (p. 15). Social workers frequently complained that their New American clients, as agencies came to identify the Soviet Jewish refugee population, were excessively demanding and overbearing, insisted on special treatment and requested more aid than agency guidelines permitted (Handelman, 1983; Stutz, 1984). Conversely, New American clients were ambivalent about the agency and the staff, and had little understanding of the nature of a voluntary agency and of professional social work. They were more likely to perceive the social work staff as government bureaucrats than as counselors, and to view the family agency as an arm of the government (Schwamm et al., 1982). They had an initial distrust of any communal agency, whether public or private, based on their negative experience with the Soviet bureaucracy. Much as the New American client disliked and distrusted government bureaucracy, it was familiar and comprehensible, whereas professional caregiving within a voluntary agency was unknown and alien. There is not even a specific word for social work in Russian, and the best translation of the word is *Vedushai*, which means guide. This is not surprising, as neither voluntary agencies nor social work as a profession existed in the Soviet Union (Brodsky, 1982; Stutz, 1984), though a variety of social work functions are performed by different government offices, trade unions and by teachers (Osborne, 1977; Handelman, 1983; Stutz, 1984). The New Americans' lack of familiarity with the American social service system together with the frequent but negative experience with Soviet bureaucracy thus produced misunderstanding and distrust. As Belozersky (1990) writes, "In a system in which an individual has very few rights and constantly is at the mercy of small and big bureaucrats, one must learn to manipulate this system to survive. When faced with survival tasks upon their arrival in the United States, many immigrants almost instinctively begin to employ the only methods they know. Because they have no frame of reference for which to understand the difference between state and voluntary agencies, any resettlement agency is seen as a continuation of the state and any caseworker as a bureaucrat who must be manipulated" (p. 126). Understanding this helped to explain cultural behavior which social workers found offensive.

The reluctance of Russians to discuss personal and emotional problems with strangers further complicated the nature of the social worker-client relationship. Russians tend to reveal problems and feelings only to close family and friends. In the repressive regime from which they came, strangers may be informers and personal revelations may lead to government punishment. "There is a strong cultural prohibition against sharing private thoughts and feelings with strangers" (Belozersky, 1990, p. 127). Furthermore, Russians are wary of mental health services and psychiatrists, as both have been punitive instruments of the state. Finally, Russian psychiatry tends to be pharmacological rather than psychodynamic in treatment approach, and thus Russians expect that treatment for emotional problems will be medication rather than counseling.

Periods of transition can be extremely stressful, and the involuntary departure from one's homeland is one of the most stressful of life's transitions, creating a state of uprootedness, vulnerability and loss (Belozersky, 1990). During such periods of life transitions, an important source of support, sustenance and assistance is the informal support system of family and friends. Jewish family service agencies quickly grew to appreciate the importance and role of the family and friendship network in the Soviet Jewish community. Soon after the first wave of refugees arrived, agencies realized that successive waves of refugees would be able to rely for assistance on family and friends already resettled. However, a key to the "collaboration between professionals and support networks in their common task of helping clients is mutual recognition of their differences . . ." (Meyer, 1985).

In the evolving division of labor, the agency handled the financial assistance program, referrals to entitlement programs and to all medical, vocational, and English language programs, as well as the responsibility for dealing with severe family or mental health problems. The informal support system of family and friends offered such assistance as meeting refugees at the airport, providing them with initial lodging, help in finding housing, and advice on everything from schools to shopping, banking and job networking. Not the least of this informal assistance was also the emotional support and reassurance provided, since verbal and emotional communication usually takes place within the family or between friends. As Belozersky (1990) states, Russians are very "warm and giving with their family and friends. Friendship is valued very highly; favors expected from and done for friends routinely would be considered an imposition by many Americans" (p. 127).

A natural collaborative and complementary partnership gradually evolved between agencies and the families and friends of New Americans, with distinct responsibilities for each. The client's natural support system emerged as an effective and generally reliable partner in the mutual goal of refugee resettlement. The agencies understood that the refugee's social network was a critically important environmental resource providing "a mutual aid system for the exchanges of instrumental assistance (such as money, child care, housing) and affective (emotional supports)" (Gitterman and Shulman, 1986, p. 7). Developing and evolving out of its own unique historical and social experiences, the New American informal support system was an effective collaborator on behalf of refugees in Soviet Jewish resettlement programs.

Unlike earlier waves of Jewish immigrants, however, the informal support network of family and friends did not translate into organized mutual aid groups. This lack is strongly regretted by all involved in Soviet Jewish resettlement activities, but it is understood as a further indication of the effect of Soviet society, in which civil organization was discouraged. Nevertheless, family and friends became an increasingly important resource, and demonstrated the efficacy of using the familiar to facilitate the challenges of the resettlement process.

Finding ways to improve mutual understanding and communication and to reduce distrust between the family service agency staff and the New American refugee population was of utmost concern from the earliest stages of the resettlement program. Educating staff about the cultural background of the client population was paramount for it could contribute to a greater understanding of the ". . . motivation behind and antecedents of demanding behavior." It might also reduce intemperate responses which can lead to a "deteriorating relationship with the client population" (Stutz, 1984, p. 188). Clients, too, needed education, particularly an introduction to the nature of American social services, and specifically an orientation to the family service agencies' resettlement programs, its objectives, policies and guidelines. To accomplish this task, many agencies organized orientation programs and/or prepared written materials in English and Russian. Several authors, reflecting on successful interventions in resettlement services, recommended that orientation programs use emigrés or staff fluent in Russian as a way to overcome cultural and linguistic barriers (Stutz, 1984; Schwamm et al., 1982).

PROFESSIONALS AND PARAPROFESSIONALS

As mentioned earlier, Jewish family service agencies, operating under the community sponsorship model of refugee resettlement, generally relied on professional social workers to deliver resettlement services. In support of professionalism in refugee services, one agency executive wrote that "professional social workers are significant in facilitating the acculturation process and are usually the most available societal role models for immigrants during the initial stage of resettlement" (p. 3). Moreover, he maintained that only a professionally trained staff can effectively juggle the complex intermingling of case manager and counselor functions required in resettlement service. "Why do we choose not to separate out the counseling aspect from the income maintenance function? Because the worker's aim is to make the refugees self-sufficient. The decision on how long to maintain them depends on professional judgments about the effort a family is putting forth" (Handelman, 1983, p. 13). From this perspective, there is a diagnostic element in resettlement which is best served by the professional social worker, such as the decision whether to extend or terminate financial assistance. This clinical approach to resettlement services reinforces professional formalism and rests on professional authority to study, diagnose, treat and prescribe.

In analyzing the social work role in refugee services, Brodsky (1982) conceptualized it as a socializing one, but, in contrast to Handelman, emphasized professional informality. In accommodating to the needs of the New American client population, Brodsky advised that social workers temper their professional stance and behave more informally, in "stark contrast to the conception of the distant, more aloof worker proposed by traditional models" (p. 15). She urged that social workers should adapt their knowledge and skills to meet the needs of this client population and bridge the cultural gap between worker and client by "offering high levels of empathy in addition to warmth and genuineness" (p. 17). She further recommended that social workers respond promptly and actively to client requests, as such concrete expressions of care tend to further the goal of establishing and advancing a trusting relationship between staff and clients.

Accepting the need for well-trained, sensitive staff, Rubin (1982) recommended that the ideal resettlement worker is one who shares a common language with the client population and has a deep appreciation for the social, political and historical background of the refugee population. At the same time, the preferred staff person should also be familiar with American social services. Rubin states that "... there is the obvious need for a highly competent staff, not only equipped with basic counseling skills but thoroughly knowledgeable and deeply empathetic to the ethnic dynamics of the refugee family–their culture, former lifestyle, family structure, language, and political systems. The ideal staff worker would be a former refugee who could speak the language and is trained as a social worker. Because this situation is rare, a second preference is for a former refugee who has the potential to benefit from skilled social work supervision" (p. 303). Rubin is thus emphasizing the idea that the ideal social worker in refugee services is one who shares with the client population the experience of migration and resettlement. The commonality of this traumatic upheaval provides what is valued in mutual aid systems where "people share relevant concerns and ideas, and begin to experience others in the same 'boat' moving through 'the rocky waters of life' . . . ." (Gitterman as quoted by Lee and Swenson, 1986, p. 362). In so doing, the trauma of migration and resettlement can be understood as a "problem in living," a "life transition" which can be overcome but is not pathological *per se*. Those who have weathered the experience become helpers and models for others who are in its throes, which gives "weight to 'normalizing' rather than 'problemizing' concerns" (Froland, 1980, p. 575). This conceptualization can be applied to resettlement services in which refugees may be understood to be "momentarily out of step" (Timberlake and Cook, 1984), and for whom the adjustment and adaptation of migration and resettlement can best be addressed by indigenous paraprofessionals. Especially in resettlement services, where utmost sensitivity to the nuances of cultural differences is paramount and where the population is generally well-functioning, professionalism and an excessive clinical orientation may reduce service effectiveness.

Some refugee programs have recognized the inappropriateness of applying a western professional conception of social work in refugee resettlement programs. In Southeast Asian refugee programs, for example, "(t)his indigenous dimension is widely recognized as an important element in the paraprofessional's value and effectiveness" (Brawley and Schindler, 1991, p. 523). These programs have been actively committed and involved in the recruitment and training of front-line service providers from among the client population. The paraprofessional Southeastern Asian resettlement workers who shared the refugee experience have been a significant bridge between cultures (Handelman, 1983). They have been role models, invaluable in helping their compatriots receive benefits and services. With training and supervision, bilingual/bicultural resettlement workers have become effective service providers bridging linguistic and cultural barriers, interpreting the agency to the clients and vice versa, and assisting clients to utilize agency as well as community services effectively (Brager, 1965; Ryan and Epstein, 1987). Based on the premise of appropriate training as a vehicle to produce a large cadre of indigenous paraprofessional resettlement workers, programs have been specifically designed to train Southeast Asian refugees for resettlement services (Ryan and Epstein, 1987).

Despite the recognition that indigenous paraprofessionals can be effective and valuable, the traditional hold of professionalism in resettlement programs for Soviet refugees delayed their acceptance as front-line service providers. As Brawley and Schindler (1991) note, ". . . there has been a failure in most parts of the world to recognize or accept the critical role played by paraprofessionals in social service delivery . . ." (p. 518). In the United States in particular, professional social work has been ambivalent at best about paraprofessionals (Brawley and Schindler, 1989). In periods of job expansion and in times when the notion of employing disadvantaged community members has been positively received, social work has supported the use of paraprofessionals. However, in times of job retrenchment, paraprofessionals have been perceived as competitors and as a threat to job security (Brawley and Schindler, 1986). Furthermore, conflicts and tensions between professionals and paraprofessionals increase when their respective job functions and roles are ambiguous and imprecisely defined (Brawley and Schindler, 1991).

The paraprofessional indigenous service provider is an unique hybrid of the professional and non-professional, emerging from a particular client group of which it is simultaneously a part and yet from which it must create and maintain some distance. As parapro-fessionals, these workers are "engaged in the provision of social care or social services to individuals, families, groups and communities but . . . do not have professional training or qualifications. They may have received some college training, participated in inservice training provided by government agencies or employers, or received no specific training for their jobs'' (Brawley and Schindler, 1991, p. 516). The indigenous paraprofessional worker stands at the interface of the formal and informal service sectors, a position containing strains and contradictions. As Froland (1980) states, ''The primary dilemmas involved in professional collaboration with informal caregivers arise out of tensions between different types of knowledge and values to which each may subscribe. The domain of professionals is usually taken to be technical skills and specialized information, while the premise of informal care is based on personal knowledge, whether through experience, background or culture'' (p. 580). Benefits in employing an indigenous staff include a shared common historical, cultural and linguistic background with the client population as well as close ties, insights and information which may facilitate rapport and enhance communication between service provider and service recipient (Brawley and Schindler, 1991). As a member of the client group who has achieved a level of acculturation, the indigenous worker can also be a socializing agent, role model and guide to the challenges of assimilating into a new society. Furthermore, the indigenous worker is usually less formal than the professional, more responsive, ''spontaneous and partisan'' (Brager, 1965, p. 36). The paraprofessional indigenous worker functions ''unencumbered'' by the professional role which is alien to the client group, gives stronger weight to ''external life circumstances than to internal factors'' and in general ''has a sense of life's meaning to the client out of their shared experience'' (Brager, 1965, p. 37).

While empathy, commonality of experience and identification with the client group may be perceived as advantages in employing indigenous workers, these same factors are also considered potential liabilities. Critics resistant to indigenous workers contend that they are inclined to overidentify and be inappropriately protective of clients. Then too they are thought to have difficulties in establishing boundaries or in setting limits. Thus, it has been suggested that in the New American program the indigenous paraprofessional might lack the resolve to implement agency policies with respect to financial assistance, housing grants, language study and job acceptance. Finally, in contrast to the professional worker, indigenous human service workers might also experience the anguish of dual loyalty, raising further question about their effectiveness as service providers.

PARAPROFESSIONALS IN A NEW AMERICAN RESETTLEMENT PROGRAM

From the very earliest days of the Soviet Jewish resettlement program, Jewish family service agencies recognized the need for a bilingual staff which would assist non-Russian speaking professional social workers to communicate with the client population. At the Boston Jewish Family and Children's Service, for example, the bilingual interpreter staff were usually not Russian. While they served a very useful function, the interpreters were also viewed with considerable dissatisfaction by the professional staff. The staff felt that the very heart of social work, the relationship between the worker and client, was being filtered through the interpreter. Sometimes it seemed that the basic relationship was not between worker and client but between interpreter and client, and that the interpreter was perceived by the client as more important than the social worker. This attitude was reinforced as interpreters accompanied clients on many critical visits outside of the agency. Interpreters received information which social workers needed to assess client progress, but only heard about later through second hand reports. Undue reliance on interpreters often had the undesired effect of interpreters dominating the interview or of staff feeling ineffective in reaching clients. Furthermore, considerable time was expended to make the social work-interpreter staff function as a team, as well as in training interpreters about the goals and methods of social work (Freed, 1988). These considerations as well as the financial burden of maintaining a large staff of interpreters and social workers contributed to a search for a more efficient use of staff.

In growing appreciation of the value of a bilingual as well as bicultural staff, the Boston Jewish Family and Children's Service gradually made the transition from a professional non-bilingual social work staff to an indigenous paraprofessional staff as the front-line service providers in its refugee resettlement program. The first step in the transition began with the use of interpreters. The second step occurred with the hiring of former clients as receptionists. This additional step was critical since the agency received numerous calls from refugee clients who spoke Russian only, and whose frustrations and hysteria mounted as they struggled to communicate on the telephone in English.

The third step in the transition occurred with the enactment of the Comprehensive and Educational Training Act (CETA) in the early 1980's which provided federal funds to human services agencies to employ non-professionals in various capacities. Several years of positive experience with the CETA program using paraprofessionals to provide resettlement services, including several bilingual/bicultural workers, further encouraged the transformation of the resettlement staff into one primarily of former refugee clients. The gradual successful deployment of a paraprofessional staff to deliver resettlement services further helped to reconceptualize the refugee resettlement as a non-clinical generic social service program.

The use of paraprofessionals required an examination and precise definition of professional and paraprofessional roles and functions in order to distinguish their respective responsibilities. Generally, paraprofessionals performed routine concrete tasks and provided emotional support, neither of which required independent decision-making or sophisticated clinical judgments. In contrast, professional responsibilities involved more complex tasks, such as "diagnostic, treatment, administrative, planning and training functions" (Brawley and Schindler, 1989, p. 100). Moreover, professional responsibility included the supervisory, administrative and clinical service of a "relatively complex nature; that is those that need more knowledge, skill and judgement than paraprofessionals typically possess, including clinical or therapeutic intervention" (Brawley and Schindler, 1986, p. 171).

As the agency gained experience with an indigenous paraprofessional staff as interpreters, receptionists, and CETA paraprofessionals providing direct services, the idea that former clients, carefully selected, could be trained to become effective service providers gained appeal and credibility. The advantages of a bilingual/bicultural paraprofessional staff were seen to outweigh the seeming disadvantages. By the end of the 1980's, former refugees were hired to staff the resettlement program, under the guidance and supervision of professional social workers. A combination of factors had converged to transform the structure of the resettlement program. These factors included "qualitative considerations" such as the recognition that "there are many functions that are particularly suitable for paraprofessionals and that some communities or client populations can be better served by indigenous front-line personnel" (Brawley and Schindler, 1989, p. 94); as well as logistic and quantitative factors, such as limited financial resources and insufficient professional staff to serve a rising caseload.

Several criteria were used in the selection of an appropriate bilingual/bicultural paraprofessional staff, similar to those applied in other refugee paraprofessional resettlement programs (Ryan and Epstein, 1987). First of these was language fluency. The language criterion was imperative as New American staff were expected to maintain records, communicate with colleagues, use the telephone to advocate for clients, and participate in staff meetings. Occasionally, New American staff were asked to make presentations to the agency board, community groups, schools or other agencies. Education was the second requirement, and all New American staff were Soviet educated university graduates, including several with professional degrees in fields such as education, psychology, engineering, medicine and library science. It was very important to hire New American staff with educational credentials, as the Soviet immigrant population is, by and large, educated and respects those with a similar education.

Furthermore, whenever possible, the staff selected had some human-service related experience in the Soviet Union. Selection and preference were given to potential employees who expressed an interest in working with people, and were strongly committed to helping their compatriots. Many New American staff prided themselves on how they had helped relatives and friends resettle. New American staff were also selected on the basis of their personal resettlement experience, and on their attitude toward the agency and its policies. Clearly, New American staff had to be comfortable with the agency objective of economic self-sufficiency, and with its policies of financial assistance and family responsibility in the resettlement process. Finally, New American staff were selected who were exemplars of successful resettlement and hence could serve as role models.

Providing appropriate training and on-going supervision is critical to the effective utilization of a paraprofessional staff (Brawley and Schindler, 1991). In Schindler and Brawley's (1987) international survey of paraprofessionals, they noted that an array of training approaches have been developed to train paraprofessionals including pre-service and in-service programs provided by employers as well as other training programs provided by educational institutions. In the case of Southeast Asian paraprofessionals, formal government sponsored training centers, institutes and programs were established to train indigenous paraprofessionals (Ryan and Epstein, 1987). However, as few indigenous paraprofessionals were used as direct service providers in resettlement programs serving Soviet Jewish refugees, there was little need for systematic training.

At the Boston Jewish Family and Children's Service it was recognized that some training and continued supervision was essential for the growing indigenous paraprofessional staff. Administrative responsibility for the refugee department was always maintained by the professional staff. Although most of the training and supervision was considered the purview of the professional staff, eventually, specific practical training was provided by experienced New American staff to new recruits. Basically the staff was trained through an apprenticeship system and a variety of in-service training modalities which included supervision, department meetings, and agency wide staff development programs. Occasionally, too, paraprofessional staff attended educational workshops and seminars relevant to the refugee experience outside the agency.

Most of the initial training focused on preparing the New American staff to perform specific routine tasks and functions. The original New American staff, which was small, received very intensive individual supervision and mentoring. With the sudden and rapid increase in the volume of cases, many additional bilingual/bicultural staff were hired, and individual supervision was superseded by group supervision and weekly unit meetings. These meetings were used to cover topics such as: orientation to the agency's philosophy of resettlement, introduction to the basics of American social service and medical care systems, and review and explanation of administrative policies and procedures. Staff meetings also became a forum for mutual support in coping with job stress and attitudes toward clients, as well as an avenue to develop and strengthen a sense of professional identity. Considerable time was devoted to professional protocol and conduct as practiced in social service agencies. Among the issues covered were the length of interviews, the locale for interviewing clients, the scheduling of client appointments, treatment of hostile clients, and maintenance of confidentiality.

As the staff became more familiar with the specific roles and tasks associated with the core resettlement service, more time was allotted to clinical issues. Clinical case conferences, led by the professional staff, allowed for review of client progress and acquisition of basic social work practice skills and techniques. Case presentations were further used to illustrate mental health concepts relevant to resettlement, for in-depth discussion of particularly difficult client issues, to assess crises and review crisis management skills. These conferences also helped the New American staff gain knowledge in assessing risk, and establishing criteria for referring clients for further professional intervention.

As part of a professional agency, an indigenous paraprofessional staff is not an isolated and static entity. They inevitably change and become professionalized through daily exposure to the agency and to the professional milieu. While professionalization is a necessary balance to overidentification and facilitates the development of ''an autonomous identity as human service workers'' (Ryan and Epstein, 1987, p. 188), there is simultaneously the apprehension that it inhibits and diminishes those very characteristics for which the indigenous workers were originally sought. Consequently, there is a tension between maintaining those positive features so frequently associated with an indigenous staff such as ''spontaneity and flexibility'' (Froland, 1980, p. 582), while providing them with professional skills which stress formality and distance. No definitive answers yet exist to the questions raised about the effect of training and institutional affiliation on the indigenous worker. According to Schindler and Brawley (1987), "workers do not have to lose their identity and effectiveness in working with their communities as a result of the training they receive" (p. 246). However, much depends on the nature of the training received and the ethos of the institutional affiliation and the trainers. In the case of the indigenous paraprofessional resettlement staff under discussion, they occasionally behaved in a bureaucratic manner towards clients or sometimes overidentified with them. In general, however, they enriched the agency by improving its ability to serve the refugee population.

The agency and the professional staff too undergo changes with the introduction of a paraprofessional staff. To avoid staff friction, there must first be clarification and precise definition of job function. Initially, this may be threatening to the professional staff as it may lead to paraprofessionals performing roles previously performed by professionals. However, it ultimately leads to a more rational use of staff with professionals performing complex jobs requiring more sophisticated clinical, administrative and supervisory knowledge and skills. Secondly, there has to be respect for and appreciation of the paraprofessionals' unique abilities and of the strengths which make them a valuable agency asset. Professional staff must be wary of undermining the work and status of paraprofessionals by condescension or by any suggestion that their function is inferior to the professional one. This is critical for staff morale, and should be demonstrated by the executive staff as well as by the rank and file. Paraprofessionals deserve admiration for the valuable contribution which they can make to the agency's capacity to serve a particular community effectively.

In the experience of the Boston Jewish Family and Children's Service, a core of competent indigenous paraprofessionals skilled in resettlement services emerged. With encouragement and financial assistance from the agency, several of them eventually entered graduate programs in social work. Upon graduation, one of this group held the position of mental health consultant to the resettlement staff. A second, very experienced indigenous resettlement worker, was promoted to a supervisory position in the resettlement program. These were positive steps and demonstrated that some upward career mobility was possible, and that an indigenous leadership was being created.

REFERENCES

Belozersky, I. (1990). New beginnings, old problems: Psychocultural frame of reference and family dynamics during the adjustment period. *Journal of Jewish Communal Service, 67*(2), 124-130.
Brager, G. (1965). The Indigenous worker: A new approach to the social work technician. *Social Work, 10*(2), 33-40.
Brawley, E. A. & Schindler, R. (1991). Strengthening professional and paraprofessional contributions to social service and social development. *British Journal of Social Work, 21*, 515-531.
Brawley, E. A. & Schindler, R. (1989). Professional-paraprofessional relationships in four countries: A comparative analysis. *International Social Work, 32*(2), 91-106.
Brawley, E.A. & Schindler, R. (1986), Paraprofessional social welfare personnel in international perspective: results of a worldwide survey. *International Social Work, 29*(2), 165-176.
Brodsky, B. (1982). Social work and the Soviet immigrant. *Migration Today, 10*, 15-20.
Brown, G. (1982). Issues in the resettlement of Indochinese refugees. *Social Casework, 63*(3), 155-159.
Freed, A. O. (1988). Interviewing through an interpreter. *Social Work, 33*(4), 315-319.
Froland, C. (1980). Formal and informal care: Discontinuities in a continuum. *Social Service Review, 54*(4), 572-587.
Freedman, R. O. (1977). The lingering impact of the Soviet system on the Soviet Jewish immigrant. In J. M. Gilson (Ed.). *The Soviet Jewish emigré* (pp. 32-58). Baltimore, MD.: Baltimore Hebrew College.
Gilson, J. M. (1977). Preface. In J.M. Gilson (Ed.). *The Soviet Jewish emigré* (pp. 7-11). Baltimore, MD.: Baltimore Hebrew College.
Gitterman, A. & Shulman, L. (1986). The life model, mutual aid, and the mediating function. In A. Gitterman & L. Shulman (Eds.). *Mutual aid groups and the life cycle* (pp. 3-23). Itasca, Il.: Peacock Press.
Haines, D. W. (1985). Refugees and the refugee program. In D.W. Haines (Ed.). *Refugees in the United States.* (pp. 3-16). Westport, Ct.: Greenwood Press.
Handelman, M. (1983). The new arrivals. *Practice Digest, 5*(4), 3-22.
Lee, J. A. B. & Swenson, C. R. (1986). The concept of mutual aid. In A. Gitterman & L. Shulman (Eds.). *Mutual aid groups and the life cycle* (pp. 361-377). Itasca, Ill.. Peacock Press.

Meyer, C.H. (1985). Social supports and social workers: collaboration or conflict? *Social Work, 30*(4), 291.

Osborne, R. J. (1977). The Soviet social environment and American contrasts. In J. M. Gilson, *The Soviet Jewish emigré* (pp. 86-98). Baltimore, MD.: Baltimore Hebrew College.

Rubin, R, S. (1982). Refugee resettlement: A unique role for family service. *Social Casework, 63*(5), 301-304.

Ryan, A. S. & Epstein, I. (1987). Mental health training for Southeast Asian refugee resettlement workers. *International Social Work, 30*(2), 185-198.

Showstack, G. L. (1990). Perspectives on the resettlement of Soviet Jews. *Journal of Jewish Communal Service, 67*(1), 66-72.

Schindler, R. & Brawley, E. A. (1987). *Social care at the front line.* New York: Tavistock Publications.

Schwamm, J., Greenstone, K. & Hoffman, H. (1982). Resettling newcomers: The case of Soviet Jewish immigration. *Arete, 7,* 25-36.

Simon, R. (1985). Soviet Jews. In D.W. Haines. *Refugees in the United States.* (pp. 181-193). Westport, Ct.: Greenwood Press.

Stutz, R. P. (1984). Resettling Soviet emigrés: How caseworkers coped. *Social Work, 9*(2), 187-188.

Timberlake, E. M. & Cook, K.O. (1984). Social work and the Vietnamese refugee. Social Work, *29*(2), 108-113.

Zukerman, K. D. (1990). The Soviet Jewish migration: Lessons for professionals. *Journal of Jewish Communal Service, 67*(2), 100-103.

TRENDS AND COMMENTARY

Planning for Pluralism:
A Report on a Chicago Agency's Efforts
on Behalf of Immigrants and Refugees

Marge Epstein
Sid L. Mohn

Founded in 1888, Travelers and Immigrants Aid of Chicago (TIA) has been providing services and advocacy on behalf of immigrants and refugees for over a century. The forbears of the current organization include Jane Addams and her League for the Protection of Immigrants. The League's work in the early 1900's in the areas of social policy research and advocacy, culturally affirming social welfare programs and immigrants rights promotion are continued today in the program portfolio of TIA.

TIA is located in the midst of the most pluralistic setting in the Midwest and one of the four most pluralistic cities in the country. The agency currently offers the following categorical and bilingual/bicultural services to immigrants and refugees from Southeast Asia, Africa, Latin America, the Middle East, and Eastern Europe.

Marge Epstein, PhD, is Assistant Professor of Social Work, Aurora University School of Social Work, Aurora, IL. Sid L. Mohn, DMin, is Executive Director of Travelers and Immigrants Aid, Chicago, IL.

Community Education Project–offers immigrants the opportunity to become legal permanent residents in the U.S. through educational programs certified to fulfill legalization requirements.

Immigrant Community Services–has a staff of attorneys and immigrant specialists to provide counseling and legal representation to immigrants. TIA assists in processing visa requests, adjusting immigrant status, becoming U.S. citizens, and in other proceedings before the Immigration and Naturalization Service.

International Refugee Center–responds to the immediate survival needs of refugees from Afghanistan, Ethiopia, Vietnam, Laos, Cambodia, and other parts of the world with a variety of programs including Refugee Resettlement and Placement program, a Refugee Case Management Service, and a Refugee Employment Service.

Marjorie Kovler Center for the Treatment of Survivors of Torture–provides psychological and physical therapy to meet the specialized needs of persons who have survived torture in their homelands, and who need help in rebuilding and restoring their lives.

Midwest Immigrant Rights Center–offers free legal assistance to indigent refugees seeking asylum in the U.S. through the services of over 170 volunteer attorneys and 70 volunteer interpreters.

Refugee Families Project–in collaboration with the Erikson Institute, helps to prepare three and four year old refugee children and their parents for school in the U.S., and enhances family ties to the community.

Refugee Mental Health Program–services include crisis intervention, individual and family counseling, assessment and mental health case management.

Refugee Substance Abuse Prevention Services–develops educational materials and community activities designed to prevent substance abuse within some of the city's refugee communities.

The Manuel Saura Center–a transitional housing program for Mariel Cubans leaving the federal correctional system.

Workplace Literacy–teaches English to immigrants, refugees and other non-English speakers by providing instruction at the job site.

In response to severe budget cuts at the federal, state and local levels, TIA held a special focus group meeting for its staff from the refugee and immigrant programs. The purpose of this meeting was threefold: to provide an assessment of refugee and immigrant needs; to assist the organization's internal planning process; and to create an agenda for influencing mainstream agencies; thereby facilitating their attentiveness and responsiveness to issues of diversity and pluralism. Below is a report from the focus group which was held in early January, 1991.

Focus group participants identified the following trends in the immigrant and refugee population:

- increase in substance abuse (particularly among survivors of torture)
- increase in family violence
- increase in the number of refugees requiring mental health interventions, (particularly Vietnamese young men who are also homeless).

Focus group participants identified the following as resource gaps within Chicago:

- affordable housing
- lack of an organized system to integrate refugees into mainstream programs
- inadequate number of staff in refugee mental health services to provide adjustment counseling, substance abuse counseling, family counseling, and intervention in more serious mental health issues
- no alcoholics anonymous groups targeted to the refugee population
- lack of programs dealing with teenage gang involvement
- a retrenchment in legal service organizations resulting in a curtailment of attorney and paralegal staff
- inadequate level of legal services for anti-deportation work.

Focus group participants identified the following observations vis a vis the assimilation process:

- People who seek out immigration services tend to have a more established social network then those who do not, i.e., they already reside in ethnic communities and have some supports in place.

- Undocumented asylum seekers tend to have a different social profile than visa applicants.
- Even though many immigrants are legalization recipients, they have become accustomed to a disempowered, undocumented status and need services leading to societal participation and empowerment.

The following recommendations were made for improving service delivery to immigrants and refugees:

- provide more advanced levels of advocacy to deal with the aftereffects of legalization
- promote citizenship efforts in an empowerment context
- fund long term case management programs to ensure continuity of care vis a vis follow-up services, especially in regard to employment
- development prevention programs for refugee communities, especially programs concerning intergenerational conflict
- develop models for mainstream providers to enhance their work with diverse cultural populations
- focus on empowerment and resources for minority women, especially around issues of health and safety
- develop volunteer network of citizens to advocate for and work with teenage gang members
- development or coordination of comprehensive refugee mental health services with linguistic and cultural relevance.

The trends and issues noted by the focus group constitute a substantial challenge requiring investment of energy and resources. State and local governments, along with private funders, need to recognize their responsibility for including long-term refugee residents in their planning and policy development. Immigrant and refugee social welfare concerns continue to be inappropriately viewed as the purview of the federal government. It is important that local agencies take a leadership role in defining the problems and responses to them. Refugee targeted programs in substance abuse, community health, employment and mental health must be embraced through a partnership of federal, state, local and private entities.

Similarly, new immigrants are still relegated to the fringes of local program commitments. Basic legal services for low income immigrants are increasingly difficult to get funded and it is even harder to find financial support for immigrant social services. Public opinion often suggests that immigrants should consider themselves fortunate to be afforded legal status and should not expect any further social assistance.

These perspectives must be changed so that we can actualize our historic rhetoric of being a nation inclusive of immigrants. In order to address the needs presented in TIA's immigrant and refugee focus group, governmental organizations and private funders must identify immigrant and refugee communities as part of their population priorities.

Commitments to pluralism must include a social welfare agenda based on domestic communities of color as well as on the social welfare needs of newly arriving and longer-term resident immigrant and refugee groups.